Managing Challenging Deformities with Arthrodesis of the Foot and Ankle

Editor

MANUEL MONTEAGUDO

FOOT AND ANKLE CLINICS

www.foot.theclinics.com

Consulting Editor
CESAR DE CESAR NETTO

December 2022 • Volume 27 • Number 4

ELSEVIER

1600 John F. Kennedy Boulevard • Suite 1800 • Philadelphia, Pennsylvania, 19103-2899

http://www.theclinics.com

FOOT AND ANKLE CLINICS Volume 27, Number 4
December 2022 ISSN 1083-7515, ISBN-978-0-323-84946-3

Editor: Megan Ashdown
Developmental Editor: Arlene B. Campos

Foot and Ankle Clinics (ISSN 1083-7515) is published quarterly by Elsevier, Inc., 360 Park Avenue South, New York, NY 10010-1710. Months of issue are March, June, September, and December. Periodicals postage paid at New York, NY, and additional mailing offices. Subscription price per year is $351.00 (US individuals), $763.00 (US institutions), $100.00 (US students), $378.00 (Canadian individuals), $786.00 (Canadian institutions), $100.00 (Canadian students), $489.00 (international individuals), $786.00 (international institutions), and $215.00 (international students). To receive student/resident rate, orders must be accompanied by name of affiliated institution, date of term, and the *signature* of program/residency coordinator on institution letterhead. Orders will be billed at individual rate until proof of status is received. Foreign air speed delivery is included in all *Clinics* subscription prices. All prices are subject to change without notice. **POSTMASTER:** Send address changes to *Foot and Ankle Clinics*, Elsevier Health Sciences Division, Subscription Customer Service, 3251 Riverport Lane, Maryland Heights, MO 63043. **Customer Service: 1-800-654-2452 (US and Canada). From outside of the United States and Canada, call 314-447-8871. Fax: 314-447-8029. E-mail: JournalsCustomerService-usa@ elsevier.com (for print support); JournalsOnlineSupport-usa@elsevier.com (for online support).**

Reprints. For copies of 100 or more, of articles in this publication, please contact the Commercial Reprints Department, Elsevier Inc., 360 Park Avenue South, New York, NY 10010-1710. Tel.: 212-633-3874; Fax: 212-633-3820; E-mail: reprints@elsevier.com.

Contributors

CONSULTING EDITOR

CESAR DE CESAR NETTO, MD, PhD
Assistant Professor, Director of the Orthopedic Functional Research Laboratory (OFIRL), Department of Orthopedics and Rehabilitation, University of Iowa, Iowa City, Iowa, USA

EDITOR

MANUEL MONTEAGUDO, MD
Orthopaedic Foot and Ankle Surgery–IOTAM, Orthopaedic Foot and Ankle Unit, Orthopaedic and Trauma Department, Hospital Universitario Quironsalud Madrid, Faculty Medicine UEM, Madrid, Spain; President Elect Spanish Foot and Ankle Society (SEMCPT), Chair Scientific Committee European Foot and Ankle Society (EFAS)

AUTHORS

AHMED KHALIL ATTIA, MD
Orthopedic Surgery and Rehabilitation Department, Orthopaedic Foot and Ankle Fellow, Penn State Milton S. Hershey Medical Center, Penn State College of Medicine, Hershey, Pennsylvania, USA

MICHAEL BRAGE, MD
Associate Professor, Department of Orthopaedics and Sports Medicine, University of Washington, Seattle, Washington, USA

DIOGO VIEIRA CARDOSO, MD
Division of Orthopaedics and Trauma Surgery, Geneva University Hospitals, Geneva, Switzerland

SAGAR CHAWLA, MD, MPH
PGY-5 Resident, Department of Orthopaedics and Sports Medicine, University of Washington, Seattle, Washington, USA

MARK E. EASLEY, MD
Department of Orthopaedic Surgery, Duke University Medical Center, Durham, North Carolina, USA

BENJAMIN J. EBBEN, MD
Foot and Ankle Surgery Fellow, Department of Orthopedic Surgery, University of Colorado School of Medicine, Aurora, Colorado, USA; Orthopedic Foot and Ankle Surgeon, Bellin Health Titletown Sports Medicine and Orthopedics, Green Bay, Wisconsin, USA

NORMAN ESPINOSA, MD
Institute for Foot and Ankle Reconstruction, FussInstitut Zurich, Zurich, Switzerland

AMANDA N. FLETCHER, MD, MSc
Resident, Department of Orthopaedic Surgery, Duke University Medical Center, Durham, North Carolina, USA

ALEXANDRE LEME GODOY-SANTOS, PhD, MD
Assistant Professor, Lab. Prof. Manlio Mario Marco Napoli, Departamento de Ortopedia e Traumatologia, Hospital das Clínicas, Faculdade de Medicina, Universidade de São Paulo, Hospital Israelita Albert Einstein, São Paulo, São Paulo, Brazil

KEITH A. HEIER, MD
Orthotexas, Dallas, Texas, USA

KENNETH J. HUNT, MD
Department of Orthopedics, University of Colorado, Aurora, Colorado, USA

JAMES A. LENDRUM, MD, MPH
Department of Orthopedics, University of Colorado, Aurora, Colorado, USA

NAJI S. MADI, MD
Foot and Ankle Surgery, Department of Orthopaedic Surgery, West Virginia University, Morgantown, West Virginia, USA

PILAR MARTÍNEZ-DE-ALBORNOZ, MD, PhD
Orthopaedic Foot and Ankle Unit, Orthopaedic and Trauma Department, Hospital Universitario Quirónsalud, Faculty Medicine UEM, Madrid, Spain

MANUEL MONTEAGUDO, MD
Orthopaedic Foot and Ankle Surgery–IOTAM, Orthopaedic Foot and Ankle Unit, Orthopaedic and Trauma Department, Hospital Universitario Quironsalud Madrid, Faculty Medicine UEM, Madrid, Spain; President Elect Spanish Foot and Ankle Society (SEMCPT), Chair Scientific Committee European Foot and Ankle Society (EFAS)

PABLO ANDRÉS CÁRDENAS MURILLO, MD
Surgical Resident, University Center for Orthopaedics, Trauma and Plastic Surgery, University Hospital Carl-Gustav Carus at TU Dresden, Dresden, Germany

MARK MYERSON, MD
Visiting Professor of Orthopedic Surgery, University of Colorado, Past President, American Orthopedic Foot and Ankle Society, Past Editor-in-Chief, *Foot and Ankle Clinics of North America*, Executive Director and Founder, Steps2Walk, Englewood, Colorado, USA

STEFAN RAMMELT, MD, PhD
Professor, Head of the Foot and Ankle Center, University Center for Orthopaedics, Trauma and Plastic Surgery, University Hospital Carl-Gustav Carus at TU Dresden, Dresden, Germany

DOV LAGUS ROSEMBERG, MD
Lab. Prof. Manlio Mario Marco Napoli, Departamento de Ortopedia e Traumatologia, Hospital das Clínicas, Faculdade de Medicina, Universidade de São Paulo, Hospital Israelita Albert Einstein, São Paulo, São Paulo, Brazil; Internacional Research Fellow of Instituto Brasil de Tecnologias da Saúde (IBTS), International Scholar at the Midwest Orthopedics at Rush (MOR), RUSH-IBTS International Fellowship Program

RAFAEL BARBAN SPOSETO, MS, MD
Lab. Prof. Manlio Mario Marco Napoli, Departamento de Ortopedia e Traumatologia, Hospital das Clínicas, Faculdade de Medicina, Universidade de São Paulo, São Paulo, São Paulo, Brazil

ANDREA VELJKOVIC, MD, FRCSC
Division of Orthopaedics and Trauma Surgery, British Columbia University, Vancouver, Canada

WOLFRAM WENZ, MD
EXPERTS FIRST Die Knochen-Docs, Heidelberg, Germany

Editorial Advisory Board

Contents

Preface: Learning Through Failure and the Way Forward   xv

Manuel Monteagudo

General Considerations About Foot and Ankle Arthrodesis. Any Way to Improve Our Results?   701

Diogo Vieira Cardoso and Andrea Veljkovic

Nonunion and adjacent joint osteoarthritis (OA) are known complications after a fusion procedure, and foot and ankle surgeons are commonly exposed to such disabling complications. Determining who is at risk of developing nonunion is essential to reducing nonunion rates and improving patient outcomes. Several evidenced-based modifiable risk factors related to adverse outcomes after foot and ankle arthrodesis have been identified. Patient-related risk factors that can be improved before surgery include smoking cessation, good diabetic control (HbAc1 <7%) and vitamin D supplementation. Intraoperatively, using less invasive techniques, avoiding joint preparation with power tools, using bone grafts or orthobiologics in more complex cases, high-risk patients, nonunion revision surgeries, and filling in bone voids at the arthrodesis site should be considered. Postoperatively, pain management with NSAIDs should be limited to a short period (<2 weeks) and avoided in high-risk patients. Furthermore, early postoperative weight-bearing has shown to be beneficial, and it does not seem to increase postoperative complications. The incidence of surrounding joint OA after foot and ankle fusion seems to increase progressively with time. Owing to its progression and high probability of being symptomatic, patients must be informed consequently, as they may require additional joint fusions, resulting in further loss of ankle/foot motion. In patients with symptomatic adjacent joint OA and unsatisfactory results after an ankle arthrodesis, conversion to total ankle arthroplasty (TAA) has become a potential option in managing these complex and challenging situations.

First Metatarsophalangeal Arthrodesis for the Failed Hallux   723

Ahmed Khalil Attia and Keith A. Heier

Hallux metatarsophalangeal joint (MTPJ) arthrodesis was first described in 1894 by Clutton, who recommended ankylosing the MTPJ to treat painful hallux valgus (HV). He used ivory pegs to stabilize the MTP joint. Surgeons over the last century have modified the procedure and added indications, including hallux rigidus, rheumatoid arthritis, and revision of failed surgeries. This article addresses many common yet challenging clinical scenarios, and a few hot topics, related to hallux MTPJ arthrodesis, including matarsus primus elevatus, severe hallux valgus, avascular necrosis, and infections. The article provides a condensed evidence-based discussion on how to manage these challenges using MTPJ arthrodesis.

Lisfranc Arthrodesis in Posttraumatic Chronic Injuries   745

Stefan Rammelt and Pablo Andrés Cárdenas Murillo

Chronic injuries at the tarsometatarsal joint represent a wide array of painful malunions ranging from isolated instability to complex three-dimensional deformities with rapid development of posttraumatic arthritis. Deformity correction and arthrodesis of the symptomatic joints leads to significant pain reduction and functional improvement provided that realignment of the anatomic axes is achieved. Arthrodesis should be limited to the first to third tarsometatarsal joints, whereas interposition arthroplasty is preferred for symptomatic arthritis of the fourth to fifth tarsometatarsal joints. For complex deformities and instability, the intercuneiform and naviculocuneiform joints may need to be included into corrective fusion.

Medial Column Fusions in Flatfoot Deformities Naviculocuneiform and Talonavicular   769

James A. Lendrum and Kenneth J. Hunt

Progressive collapsing foot deformity (PCFD; commonly referred to as flatfoot deformity) is a complex condition classically characterized by hindfoot valgus, midfoot abduction, and forefoot varus. Medial column arthrodesis can be used to reliably correct severe, arthritic, and unstable PCFD involving the medial column. Although both naviculocuneiform arthrodesis and talonavicular arthrodesis have their own indications, patient selection and careful radiographic and clinical assessment are crucial for any medial column arthrodesis. Herein, the authors discuss the indications for medial column arthrodesis procedures, outcomes as reported in the literature, and several case examples using medial column arthrodesis in deformity correction.

Management of the Subtalar Joint Following Calcaneal Fracture Malunion   787

Benjamin J. Ebben and Mark Myerson

Subtalar joint arthrosis is common following intra-articular calcaneus fractures. The appropriate management of pain secondary to posttraumatic arthritis depends on the status of the remaining posterior facet articular cartilage, the magnitude of any residual joint displacement and distortions in the overall morphology of the calcaneus. In select circumstances, joint-preserving surgical techniques may be considered including lateral wall exostectomy, far lateral posterior facet joint debridement, and intra-articular osteotomies. When the subtalar joint is not salvageable, some form of arthrodesis procedure is pursued. Occasionally, an extra-articular osteotomy may be necessary in combination with arthrodesis to correct deformity.

Double and Triple Tarsal Fusions in the Severe Rigid Flatfoot Deformity   805

Naji S. Madi, Amanda N. Fletcher, and Mark E. Easley

A flatfoot deformity is a multiplanar foot deformity characterized by forefoot abduction and supination and hindfoot valgus. With progressive pathology, a rigid deformity may develop. In the setting of a rigid deformity, the appropriate procedure to use is not without controversy. The extent of joints to involve in the arthrodesis depends on the ability to obtain a plantigrade foot. Both double and triple arthrodesis have been suggested. Care must be taken to avoid lateral column shortening and loss of foot reduction when fusing the CC joint. The concerns about lateral skin breakdown led some surgeons to describe a single medial incision for a triple or modified double arthrodesis. The necessity of bone grafting has been controversial. Implant selection is essential to achieve solid stabilization of the arthrodesis sites. To decrease the risk of overcorrection and malunion, the surgeon should be familiar with the hindfoot biomechanics and generate, based on the clinical examination and imaging, a meticulous preoperative plan to address and balance both the soft tissue and bony deformity.

Double and Triple Tarsal Fusions in the Complex Cavovarus Foot   819

Wolfram Wenz

The cavovarus (cavus) foot is one of the most perplexing and challenging of all foot deformities and may prove to be one of the most difficult conditions to treat. This deformity is characterized by increased plantar flexion of the forefoot and midfoot in relation to the hindfoot resulting in high foot arch. Because cavus foot rarely occurs in an isolated form, the term "cavus foot" rather describes a part of a complex multiplanar foot deformity. Because the underlying disease is mostly neurogenic characterized by muscle imbalance in almost every case a combined bony and soft tissue surgery is inevitable.

Arthrodesis in the Deformed Charcot Foot   835

Dov Lagus Rosemberg, Rafael Barban Sposeto, and Alexandre Leme Godoy-Santos

Charcot neuroarthropathy (CN) is a systemic disease that causes fractures, dislocations, and deformities involving the foot and ankle, resulting in substantial risk of ulceration, infection, and function loss. Early recognition and prevention of collapsing foot and ankle are still the best options for the management of patients with diabetic CN. For a successful arthrodesis procedure, the principles of adequate joint preparation, deformity correction, and soft tissue protection and care are essentials, associated with robust fixation (internal and/or external), use of different biological graft options in segmental losses, and prolonged off-loading.

Tibiotalocalcaneal Arthrodesis in Severe Hindfoot Deformities   847

Pilar Martínez-de-Albornoz and Manuel Monteagudo

Tibiotalocalcaneal arthrodesis is the most common and reliable procedure in the treatment of patients with end stage ankle arthritis combined with severe deformity. Many patients present with difficult previous sequelae that include nonunion, malunion, broken implants, vascular deficiencies, skin problems or a combination of the previous. TTCA with grafting allows for the preservation of the limb in more than 80% of cases. The studies presented in this paper have a considerable wide array of different scenarios that present a persuasive pattern towards considering TTC with grafting and nail or plate fixation as a good salvage procedure.

Ankle Arthrodesis in Crippled Cases   867

Norman Espinosa

> The current article provides an algorithm of how to approach crippled ankle by ankle arthrodesis. There is no standard pathology or treatment present, which makes the diagnosis but also surgical correction complex. A surgeon who faces this kind of deformities needs to be skilled and well familiar with the full setting of the foot and ankle armamentarium.

Pantalar Arthrodesis   883

Sagar Chawla and Michael Brage

> A triple arthrodesis is comprised of subtalar, talonavicular, and calcaneocuboid joints arthrodesis. A pantalar arthrodesis is triple arthrodesis combined with tibiotalar arthrodesis. The goal of the procedure is to obtain a correction of deformity and achieve a plantigrade, functional, painless, stable, weightbearing foot that can be used to ambulate. This is done by creating an osseous continuity across the ankle, subtalar, and talonavicular, and calcaneocuboid joints. There are several approaches and fixation strategies that result in successful clinical union and should be chosen to match the clinical situation. Modern techniques result in high rates of union and pain relief.

FOOT AND ANKLE CLINICS

FORTHCOMING ISSUES

MARCH 2023
Applied Translational Research in Foot and Ankle Surgery
Don Anderson, *Editor*

JUNE 2023
Advanced Imaging in Foot and Ankle
Jan Fritz, *Editor*

September 2023
Complexities Involving the Ankle Sprain
Alexandre Godoy-Santos, *Editor*

RECENT ISSUES

September 2022
The Diabetic Foot
Fabian Krause, *Editor*

JUNE 2022
Managing Complications of Foot and Ankle Surgery
Scott Ellis, *Editor*

MARCH 2022
Alternatives to Ankle Joint Replacement
Woo-Chun Lee, *Editor*

RELATED SERIES

Orthopedic Clinics
Clinics in Sports Medicine
Physical Medicine and Rehabilitation Clinics

THE CLINICS ARE NOW AVAILABLE ONLINE!
Access your subscription at:
www.theclinics.com

Preface

Learning Through Failure and the Way Forward

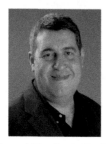

Manuel Monteagudo, MD
Editor

It is a big honor to be the guest editor for this issue of *Foot and Ankle Clinics of North America*. Being guest editor is harder than I ever thought and more rewarding than I could have ever imagined. Orthopedic Foot and Ankle Surgery has advanced dramatically over the last years, notably due to new procedures that have also given rise to new complex scenarios for revision surgery. The additional surgical demands presented by complex deformities after failed surgeries have stimulated the adage that "necessity is the mother of invention". Complex deformities are usually the result of complex cases with suboptimal results and are disheartening to surgeons and devastating for our patients. Sometimes, good index surgery can be negated by noncompliant patients and metabolic disorders, but some other times the type of surgery was not the best approach for the problem, it was not well executed, or both. Revisional surgery not only challenges surgical skills but also tests the surgeon's ability to interact with patients, industry, and other colleagues/specialists, and to plan for the best implants and biologics to get things right. Although living in an era of joint-preserving surgery, severe deformity and extensive joint damage oblige us to perform big deformity corrections with arthrodesis. A big problem needs a big hammer (and this issue). The surgeon needs to explain to a patient why a previous surgery failed and why the new salvage procedure with an arthrodesis might work. Ultimately, the patient's needs must be placed at the center of this decision-making process. Sometimes the best option is to not operate at all but, when it comes to surgery, sometimes the only alternative to complex reconstruction with arthrodesis is an amputation.

The ability and capacity to successfully address complications and failed surgeries are not easily learned from literature but rather are an art that we all learn from our mentors and colleagues, as well as from experience through our own successes and failures. I expect the articles you are about to read will be helpful when facing challenging cases and stimulate your imagination. Our own "road of failure" should not cultivate a

Foot Ankle Clin N Am 27 (2022) xv–xvi
https://doi.org/10.1016/j.fcl.2022.09.001
1083-7515/22/© 2022 Published by Elsevier Inc.

foot.theclinics.com

culture of blame but rather motivate and inspire us to drive improvement into our surgical practice. I am confident that cultural and cognitive diversity from the different expert authors in this issue will lead you to the most suitable way forward whenever you are planning a complex arthrodesis for a complex unconventional case.

The issue you have ahead would have not been possible without my mentor and friend Mark Myerson offering me to coordinate this issue and without the Consulting Editor, Cesar de Cesar Netto, inspiring me through the process of editing with his passion in steering *Foot and Ankle Clinics of North America* from strength to strength. They both have given me the opportunity to gather an outstanding group of colleagues and friends. I am privileged to present authors with wide experience in complex arthrodesis who provide us with examples of severe foot and ankle deformities, highlighting tips and tricks that are the result of years of learning through failure and expertise. They have done a tremendous job of giving rational approaches to complex deformities with arthrodesis and simplifying the complex so that their clear ideas enter our brains quicker and stay there longer. It has been an honor to work with each of them, and I have learned from them all. This issue would not have been possible without the help and support from Arlene, Megan, and all the Elsevier team in the backstage. My gratitude for their editorial help, keen insight, and ongoing support that have been essential to bring all articles to production and to you.

I wish you happy reading!

Manuel Monteagudo, MD
Orthopaedic Foot and Ankle Surgery–IOTAM
Hospital Universitario Quironsalud
Faculty Medicine UEM
Madrid, Spain

E-mail address:
mmontyr@yahoo.com

General Considerations About Foot and Ankle Arthrodesis. Any Way to Improve Our Results?

Diogo Vieira Cardoso, MD[a],*, Andrea Veljkovic, MD, FRCSC[b]

KEYWORDS

- Arthrodesis • Nonunion risk factors • Ankle arthrodesis • Ankle osteoarthritis
- Foot arthrodesis

KEY POINTS

- A successful joint fusion depends on a complex relationship of several factors, such as patient-related factors, intraoperative, and postoperative factors.
- With smoking cessation, good diabetic control (HbAc1 <7%) and vitamin D supplementation before the procedure, the outcomes after foot and ankle arthrodesis can be improved.
- Patient outcomes and postoperative complications can be improved by using less invasive techniques, even in the presence of more severe deformities.
- Using bone grafts in more complex cases, high-risk patients, nonunion revision surgeries, and filling in bone voids at the arthrodesis site, should be considered.
- The incidence of surrounding joint osteoarthritis after foot and ankle fusion seems to increase progressively with time. Owing to its progression and high probability of being symptomatic, patients must be informed consequently, as they may require additional joint fusions, resulting in further loss of ankle/foot motion.

INTRODUCTION

The etymology of the word arthrodesis shows that it originated from *arthro(English)* + *"dese,"* from the Greek meaning binding together.[1] The first known use of arthrodesis was in 1888, suggesting that surgeons for thousands of years have performed this procedure.[1] Historically, its main indication was to treat painful osteoarthritis, but with the arrival of arthroplasty, joint arthrodesis for osteoarthritis

Funded by: SWISS2021.
[a] Division of Orthopaedics and Trauma Surgery, Geneva University Hospitals, Rue Gabrielle-Perret-Gentil 4, Geneva 1205, Switzerland; [b] Division of Orthopaedics and Trauma Surgery, British Columbia University, Vancouver, Canada
* Corresponding author.
E-mail address: diogo.vieiracardoso@hcuge.ch

has been decreasing and almost not performed, namely in hip and knee. However, in foot and ankle surgery, arthrodesis procedures remain an essential treatment tool for foot and ankle surgeons, as joint fusions are performed to treat a variety of pathologies from an isolated Hallux Rigidus to a complex midfoot/hindfoot deformity, tendon dysfunction, and neurologic foot problems.[2–4]

Nonunion and adjacent joint osteoarthritis are known complications after a fusion procedure, and foot and ankle surgeons are commonly exposed to such disabling complications. Nonunion has been associated with high patient morbidity and increased health costs, which justifies the resources and research focused on improving fusion rates in elective fusion procedures.[2] As a result, reducing nonunion rates has been a goal in foot and ankle surgery.[2] Nonunion rates of standard foot and ankle arthrodesis are illustrated in **Table 1**.

Determining who is at risk of developing nonunion is essential to reducing nonunion rates and improving patient outcomes. Several patient-related risk factors such as smoking and diabetes have been strongly associated with nonunion in foot and ankle surgery.[5–7] However, a successful bony fusion depends on a more complex relationship of several factors other than patients' comorbidities as several technical and mechanical factors have also been related determinants for nonunion development.[8]

This article exposes the most frequent factors related to nonunion and adjacent joint osteoarthritis after foot and ankle arthrodesis procedures. It provides the insight and necessary knowledge to properly inform patients about potential adverse outcomes and how to improve outcomes after foot and ankle arthrodesis. With this in mind, we have divided these factors into 3 main categories according to their relationship with the surgery into (1) preoperative; (2) intraoperative; (3) postoperative (**Table 2**).

Preoperative Factors

This group includes all the modifiable risk factors in patients who could benefit from focused preoperative education and treatment modification to improve patient outcomes and decrease the nonunion rate. Most of these risk factors are related to the patient's comorbidities or health habits.

Smoking

The effect of smoking on foot and ankle procedures is likely to be more pronounced when compared with other orthopedic surgical subspecialties. Peripherally, nicotine decreases prostacyclin, leading to vasoconstriction and tissue hypoperfusion.[9] Nicotine also potentiates platelet adhesion resulting in microvascular clot formation.[9,10] Carbon monoxide in cigarette smoke binds to hemoglobin and shifts the oxygen

Table 1	
Nonunion rates in common arthrodesis performed in foot and ankle surgery	
Fusion Procedure	Non-union Rates (%)
Ankle arthrodesis	3%–11%[2]
Subtalar arthrodesis	10%–23%[111–113]
Talonavicular arthrodesis	4%–7%[3]
Midfoot arthrodesis	7%–13%[4,114]
First TMT arthrodesis	2%–10%[64]
First MTP arthrodesis	3%–5%[115,116]

Abbreviations: MTP, metatarsophalangeal; TMT, tarsometatarsal.

Table 2 Modifiable risk factors for adverse outcomes after foot and ankle arthrodesis according to the operative period	
Preoperative	• Smoking • Diabetes • BMI • Vitamin D levels • Medications (Corticosteroids)
Intraoperative	• Open surgery vs less invasive procedures • Joint alignment • Method for joint preparation • Interfragmentary gap • Use or not use bone graft and which type
Postoperative	• NSAID medication • Early vs delayed weight bearing • Surrounding joint OA and additional fusions

dissociation curve to the left, which causes oxygen dissociation from hemoglobin and further tissue hypoperfusion.[9] In addition, there is evidence showing an association between smoking and low bone mineral density, delayed fracture union, and implant failure.[10] A recent review of literature involving 91 studies assessing the effect of smoking in trauma and elective foot and ankle procedures concluded that it seems to be a significantly increased risk of nonunion in ankle, hindfoot and midfoot arthrodesis performed in smokers.[11] The odds ratio of smokers in hindfoot and midfoot arthrodesis nonunions was reported as 3.9 and 8.5, respectively. Moreover, major postoperative complications such as deep infections and wound healing problems were significantly higher in smokers. In another study, Thevendran and colleagues[12] completed a review on the risks of nonunion in foot and ankle arthrodesis. Although all included studies were level III and IV evidence, they concluded that there was enough evidence to support a grade B recommendation on smoking as a risk factor for nonunion in foot and ankle fusions.

In clinical practice, patients are often requested to stop or reduce tobacco smoking to improve postoperative outcomes. It has been reported that self-reporting of tobacco use is underestimated by up to 25% of actual smoking status.[13] Thus, on occasions, it can be helpful to determine the right level of tobacco smoking. The 2 most common methods of smoking assessment currently in use are exhaled carbon monoxide and saliva cotinine measurement. Passive smokers usually have cotinine concentrations in saliva below 5 ng/ml. Levels between 10 and 100 ng/mL may result from infrequent active smoking and levels >100 ng/mL from regular active smoking.[14]

It is known that immune and pulmonary function improves after smoking cessation.[15] Moreover, a comparative level- I study has shown that smoking cessation for 4 weeks preoperatively reduced the risk of postoperative complications comparable to nonsmoking patients.[16,17] Although evidence is quite limited, it seems that smoking has a significant negative impact on foot and ankle fusion procedures outcomes. Thus, it is recommended that active smokers decrease or stop smoking in the perioperative period (4 weeks ideally) of a surgical procedure.

Obesity

In orthopedic surgery, obesity has often been associated with increased postoperative complications, such as wound healing problems and fracture nonunion.[18–21] Obese patients may encounter cast and brace fitting challenges and may have difficulty maintaining non–weight-bearing postoperatively. These circumstances can compromise the fixation and increase the mechanical load on the implant's fusion site, leading to unwanted motion at the arthrodesis. The available literature assessing the impact of BMI on the outcome of arthrodesis procedures is exceptionally scarce or inexistent. However, studies assessing the outcomes of femur and proximal tibial realignment osteotomies have shown significantly higher rates of nonunion in obese patients.[22,23] Nevertheless, there is no evidence supporting obesity as an independent risk factor for arthrodesis nonunion in the foot and ankle field.

Diabetes

The pathophysiology of diabetic bone healing has been studied extensively in animal and clinical models.[24] Through several mechanisms such as sustained hyperglycemia and increased the activation of proinflammatory factors, diabetes disrupts the homeostasis between osteoblasts and osteoclasts' activity.[25] In the process of fracture healing, the reparative stage involves the formation of cartilage during endochondral bone formation by chondrocytes and bone production by osteoblasts. Moreover, angiogenesis enhances cartilage transition into bone. Impaired osteoclasts and osteoblasts function to organize bone into its final form, and states of hyperglycemia and insulin insufficiency are proposed mechanisms that alter chondrocyte and osteoblast apoptosis, interfering with bone healing.[24] Diabetes increases blood viscosity and is associated with tissue hypoxia.[26] In addition to affecting the angiogenesis process, tissue hypoxia slows inflammatory responses, thereby altering wound healing and increasing the risk of infection, particularly in the lower extremity.[25,26]

The negative impact of diabetes on fracture healing is widely supported. For example, a recent systematic review comparing rates of adverse healing outcomes in patients with diabetes versus nondiabetes following surgical treatment of a lower extremity fracture concluded that patients with diabetes are at a significantly higher risk of nonunion (approximately six times) especially in fractures involving the lower leg.[25] A retrospective comparative study assessing the outcomes of ankle and hindfoot fusions in patients with and without diabetes found that the overall rate of postoperative complications (infection and nonunion) was significantly higher in patients with diabetes (45% vs 22%, $P < .005$).[27] Moreover, patients with diabetes had a two times higher likelihood of developing a nonunion when compared with patients with nondiabetes.

It is well known that patients with poorly controlled diabetes are more likely to experience complications of diabetes, such as neuropathy, foot ulcer, and Charcot foot condition.[28] Poorly controlled glucose (Hgb A1c greater than or equal to 7%) in patients with diabetes has been associated with two- and five-times higher likelihood of developing a postoperative nonunion and infection, respectively.[27,29]

There is fair evidence supporting diabetes as a risk factor for postoperative complications after foot and ankle arthrodesis. In addition, poorly controlled glucose with Hgb A1c superior to 7% seems to increase complications incidence in patients with diabetes. Therefore, close glycemic control and multidisciplinary diabetic consultation are recommended before any foot and ankle surgery.

Vitamin D

Vitamin D is essential in maintaining bone health through calcium and phosphate metabolism regulation. When vitamin D levels are low, the absorption of calcium and phosphate in the intestine decreases, causing an increase in parathyroid hormone, which results in increased osteoclastic activity.[30] Hypovitaminosis D is not rare as we might think. Vitamin D levels have been reported as low in 70% of orthopedic patients and as severely low in 22% of patients undergoing elective foot and ankle procedures.[31]

Inadequate sun exposure, gastrointestinal malabsorption syndromes, and renal failure are frequent causes of insufficient levels of vitamin D. Current evidence about the role of vitamin D on foot and ankle conditions are limited owing to the anecdotic number of high-level evidence studies. One study comparing vitamin D levels between patients with ankle fractures and patients with ankle sprains has shown significantly lower vitamin D levels in the ankle fracture group.[32] Another case-control retrospective study compared 29 patients with nonunion following elective foot and ankle reconstruction with a control group of 29 patients with a successful union.[33] They assessed the prevalence of modifiable risk factors for nonunion and found statistically significant lower vitamin D levels in the nonunion group. Moreover, patients with vitamin D deficiency or insufficiency were 8.1 times more likely to experience nonunion.

Animal models suggest that vitamin D supplementation facilitates fracture healing.[30] In addition, a randomized clinical trial after proximal humerus fracture in humans showed increased fracture callus formation with vitamin D and calcium supplementation compared with placebo.[34] For an adult, vitamin D levels of 75 mmol/L or superior are considered as normal or sufficient to maintain bone health, and the recommended daily intake of vitamin D for healthy individuals is 600 IU (international units) for those younger than 70 and 800 IU after age 71.[33]

Based on the limited evidence, hypovitaminosis D in foot and ankle patients is a frequent condition. Therefore, screening and hypovitaminosis D treatment supplementation is recommended as the benefits seem to outweigh the drawbacks, and outcomes of the arthrodesis procedure may be improved as a result.

Patient Medications

Several medications used to treat chronic medical conditions, especially those commonly prescribed to treat rheumatologic and inflammatory diseases have come under consideration for their theoretical ability to alter the early inflammatory pathway and the later molecular environment involved in bone and wound healing, thereby potentially resulting in undesirable postoperative complications. For example, animal studies have shown that long-term use of corticosteroids leads to osteoblast apoptosis, osteocyte apoptosis, and inhibition of osteoblastogenesis, resulting in decreased bone density and callus formation.[35,36] In an experimental model of posterolateral lumbar spinal arthrodesis in rabbits, dexamethasone administration inhibited graft incorporation and increased rates of nonunion.[37] Although the inhibitory effect of corticosteroids on bone healing seems logical, these results have been found primarily in animal studies.

For other drugs, such as methotrexate, the effect on bone healing seems to be dose-related as a low dose of methotrexate did not affect the early process of endochondral bone formation in experimental studies.[38] Regarding wound healing, in vitro and experimental animal studies suggest that methotrexate can adversely affect wound healing, whilst the clinical studies show that lose-dose methotrexate is safe and does not affect the incidence of postoperative wound complications.[39]

The effect on bone healing of oncologic drugs has been investigated. The antiproliferative and cytotoxic properties of chemotherapeutic agents seem to alter neovasculogenesis, proper callus formation, and host bone-allograft incorporation resulting in higher nonunion rates.[40] Quinolones have been associated with decreased chondrocyte number, abnormalities in cartilage morphology and impaired fracture healing in rats.[41]

Today's knowledge of the effect of several drugs on bone healing is characterized by inconclusive and controversial results from several animal models. However, evidence suggests that some pharmacologic agents can be detrimental to bone healing and affect patient's outcome following arthrodesis surgery. Considering this, physicians should inquire about patients' medications, perform necessary adjustments, and, perhaps, consider delaying surgery whenever indicated.

Intraoperative Factors

This group includes all the modifiable factors during the surgical procedure. Most of them are related to surgical techniques and surgeons' choices.

Open vs. arthroscopic surgery: does it matter?

Foot and ankle joint arthrodesis have been traditionally performed through open techniques. The small size of most joints has been the main drawback of using less invasive techniques such as arthroscopy. However, improved instrumentation and more significant experience have facilitated the development of new and less invasive approaches. As a result, arthroscopic arthrodesis procedures have gained increasing popularity among foot and ankle surgeons. Owing to their minimally invasive nature, arthroscopic techniques provide specific benefits: minimal soft tissue damage with less blood supply disruption, improved intra-articular visualization, minimal bone resection, improved fusion surface preparation, reduced postoperative pain, diminished wound healing complications, and a superior cosmetic result.[42–44] The majority of studies comparing open versus arthroscopic joint fusion assess the ankle and subtalar joints. A recent systematic review compared the outcome of arthroscopic ankle fusion in 303 patients with open ankle arthrodesis in 214 patients.[45] Only ankle arthrodesis for ankle osteoarthritis was included. Overall, the arthroscopic group had significantly higher fusion rates, less blood loss, shorter tourniquet times, shorter length of hospitalization, and better recovery at 1 year. Another multicentric comparative study found shorter length of hospitalization and significantly better outcomes one and 2 years after arthroscopic ankle fusion.[46] Moreover, arthroscopic ankle fusion has been associated with less postoperative pain and fewer complications such as wound healing problems and nerve injury.[47,48] In patients at high risk of postoperative complications, arthroscopic fusion significantly decreased major surgical-site-infections.[49]

The use of arthroscopic arthrodesis in patients with more severe angular deformities has been a debatable question. Whereas initially it was considered suitable only for minimally deformed arthritic ankles, evidence shows that similar good results can be obtained in more severe deformities.[50,51] Issac and colleagues compared the results of arthroscopic and open ankle fusions in patients with less than 15° of coronal plane angulation versus patients with more than 15° of coronal plane deformity.[52] They found equal good deformity correction with both techniques, and the degree of deformity did not adversely affect the outcome of arthroscopic ankle arthrodesis compared with an open procedure. Moreover, significantly higher rates of nonunion were observed in patients with more than 15° of deformity treated with open techniques. An example of a severe ankle valgus ball and socket deformity treated with arthroscopic ankle fusion is illustrated in **Fig. 1**.

Although there is strong evidence supporting the benefits of arthroscopic over open techniques in ankle arthrodesis, the available evidence comparing both procedures in other foot joints is still limited. A recent prospective multicenter randomized controlled trial compared the results of open posterior subtalar fusion in 28 patients with posterior arthroscopic subtalar arthrodesis (PASTA) in 28 patients.[53] Union time (9.4 vs 12.8 weeks) and recovery time (time to return to activities of daily living [8.4 vs 10.8 weeks]) were significantly shorter with PASTA than with the open technique. Other outcomes, including tourniquet time (55.8 vs 67.2 min), union rate (96.3% vs 100%), and

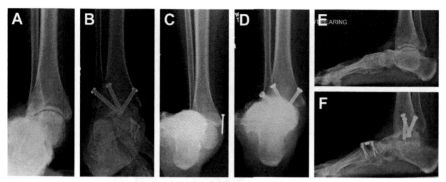

Fig. 1. Pre and postoperative imaging of a 34-year-old patient with severe ankle valgus ball and socket deformity treated with arthroscopic ankle fusion. (*A*) Preoperative weight-bearing AP ankle radiograph. (*B*) Postoperative weight-bearing AP ankle radiograph. (*C*) Preoperative weight-bearing hindfoot view. (*D*) Postoperative weight-bearing hindfoot view. radiograph. (*E*) Preoperative weight-bearing lateral ankle radiograph. (*F*) Postoperative weight-bearing lateral ankle radiograph.

complication rate, were not significantly different between the techniques. Similar results were observed by Rungprai and colleagues in another retrospective comparative study with 57 patients in the open group and 64 patients in the arthroscopic group.[54-] Because of their size and limited motion, midfoot joints were traditionally fused with open techniques. However, with new techniques, arthroscopic arthrodesis of midfoot joints such as the talonavicular, calcaneocuboid, and first TMT joint is becoming more frequent.[55–57] A recent retrospective study compared the radiographic correction and complication rates between 47 patients treated with arthroscopic first TMT fusion and 44 patients treated with open first TMT fusion for hallux valgus deformity.[57] Both techniques showed comparable good to excellent deformity correction. However, wound complications and non-union rates trended higher in the open group (4 vs 0, P=.051).

Based on the available evidence, it seems that patient outcomes and postoperative complications can be improved by using less invasive techniques, even in the presence of more severe deformities.

Malalignment

The position of each lower extremity joint intimately affects adjacent joint function as well as whole-limb performance. For instance, ankle fusion in the equinus position may result in accelerated subtalar changes and has been associated with recurvatum and laxity of the medial collateral ligament at the knee caused by back-kneeing and externally rotating the limb and stance.[58] Excessive hindfoot varus is often mal tolerated as can lead to excessive lateral column loading.[59] In triple hindfoot arthrodesis, residual hindfoot valgus and forefoot supination may cause subfibular impingement and deltoid failure resulting in ankle valgus.[60] An example of an ankle valgus after a triple arthrodesis with residual hindfoot valgus and forefoot supination malalignment is illustrated in **Fig. 2**.

Nevertheless, some degree of malalignment can be beneficial and improve outcomes in certain type of patients. For example, posterior displacement of the talus under the tibia is thought to reduce distal tibial pain and midfoot stress. This posterior displacement, combined with external rotation of 5 to 10°, reduces the foot lever arm and the tendency of the proximal joints to rotate externally during gait.[59] Thus,

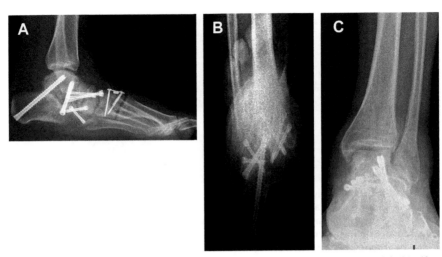

Fig. 2. Postoperative weight-bearing foot and ankle radiographs showing a triple hindfoot fusion with residual hindfoot valgus and inadequate plantar flexion of the first ray resulting in deltoid ligament insufficiency and ankle valgus. (*A*) Postoperative lateral foot view showing absence of first ray plantar flexion. (*B*) Postoperative hindfoot view showing residual hindfoot valgus. (*C*) Postoperative ankle view showing nonconcentric valgus ankle.

ankle fusion with slight posterior displacement of the talus may improve outcomes in patients presenting with concomitant midfoot degeneration. When performing first tarsometatarsal joint fusion for midfoot osteoarthritis and hallux valgus deformity in patients with early features of progressive collapsing foot deformity, surgeons should consider increasing first ray plantar flexion to stabilize the medial column, correct hindfoot alignment, and bring the foot to a plantigrade position that protects the whole foot construction and ankle joint.[61]

Joint preparation

Joint preparation can be performed through several different techniques. Tools such as osteotomes, curettes, and rongers are frequently used to remove the cartilage. Because thorough joint preparation with these tools can be time-consuming, power tools such as saws, burrs, and reamers have been developed and adapted to facilitate foot and ankle joint arthrodesis procedures. However, the use of power tools in joint preparation has several nonnegligible drawbacks. Firstly, they can be a source of thermal bone necrosis, as higher burr and reamer speed causes an increase in bone temperature.[62] One systematic review comparing the effect of joint preparing in first metatarsophalangeal arthrodesis found higher rates of nonunion when power tools are used for cartilage removal.[63] Therefore, temperature control with saline solution irrigation should be applied when high-velocity surface preparation methods are used. Secondly, joint preparation with power tools can cause excessive subchondral bone removal with secondary joint and bone shortening.[64] This concerns more mid and forefoot arthrodesis procedures such as tarsometatarsal joint arthrodesis as excessive metatarsal shortening can lead to postoperative metatarsalgia.[61] Using saw cuts in Lapidus arthrodesis has been associated with excessive first ray shortening compared with more conservative methods such as curettes.[65]Once the cartilage is removed, sequentially drilling multiple holes in bone is often used to aid fusion.

However, drilling induces a significant amount of heat and accumulates after multiple passes, resulting in thermal osteonecrosis and detrimental to patient outcomes.[66] Although available evidence does not support one specific standard preparation method, the surgeon must be aware of the risks when using high-velocity tools for joint preparation, and actions to mitigate such risks should be employed. Several factors, such as tool selection and geometry, the time interval between passes, and drilling technic, can be modified to reduce heat-related bone injuries during joint preparation.[66,67] Ideally, surgeons should: use twist drills rather than Kirschner wires to improve bone chips evacuation; prefer drill bits of small diameter (<2.0 mm) to decrease bone contact; decrease the time interval between passes to reduces the total heat exposure time; optimize the drilling sequence and technic applying more perpendicular drill angles; perform irrigation and bone chips evacuation regularly.

Interfragmentary bone gap
The notion that increasing the interfragmentary gap would impair bone healing and alter the outcome is strongly supported mainly by animal studies.[68,69] It has been shown that a higher bone gap is associated with delayed bone healing, decreased callus and bone volume formation.[68] Although evidence on animal studies seems to be unanimous, there is a paucity in human studies, mainly owing to the difficulties in isolating bone gap as the only risk factor for bone healing. Perhaps, the only study assessing the role of poor bone apposition and the presence of bone gaps in achieving fusion in foot and ankle arthrodesis involving human subjects has been performed by DiGiovanni et al.[70] In their level- II study, the authors evaluated the importance of adequate graft material (defined as graft material filling >50% of the gap between bones) to obtain fusion in hindfoot and ankle arthrodesis. In their results, 81% of joints with good graft fill were successfully fused at 24 weeks compared with only 21% without adequate graft fill ($P < .001$). Furthermore, the OR for successful fusion with or without adequate graft fill did not differ significantly when stratified by joint type, the number of joints fused, sex, age, BMI, diabetes, or smoking status. Joints that had undergone a previous operation (other than fusion) at a fusion site had a significantly lower OR of successful fusion, although having good graft fill was still beneficial for fusion. They concluded an association between the amount of graft material, adequate graft filling, and successful ankle and hindfoot arthrodesis. Therefore, when a surgeon can eliminate bone-to-bone gaps in any joint intended for fusion, whether via the use of autograft or similar orthobiological, such a joint has a significantly better chance of ultimately achieving fusion.

Bone graft: use or not use?
Using bone graft to improve outcomes and achieve fusion in arthrodesis surgeries is a common procedure in foot and ankle surgery. However, the question of whether bone graft should be performed in primary arthrodesis procedures, in high-risk patients, or only in nonunion revision surgeries is still unanswered. Despite extensive literature citing the use of autograft or suitable alternatives to promote fusion in ankle and hindfoot arthrodesis, there is a remarkable paucity of level-I or II studies directly comparing rates of union with and without the use of graft material. In a recent systematic review including 27 studies, Heifner and colleagues assessed the role of bone grafting on fusion rates in primary open ankle arthrodesis.[71] Their results showed equivalent fusion rates between the graft and no graft group, and the authors conclude that the routine use of bone graft may not be needed in primary ankle arthrodesis in low-risk patients. However, the evidence seems to suggest the opposite regarding arthrodesis involving other foot joints.[72] Buda and colleagues assessed the effect of

bone grafting on union rates in 88 patients undergoing primary tarsometatarsal arthrodesis for tarsometatarsal osteoarthritis and concluded that the use of autologous bone grafting significantly reduced the risk of nonunion. Thus, for primary tarsometatarsal joint arthrodesis, the use of bone graft can be advantageous in improving outcomes.

The decision to use a bone graft or any orthobiologics in arthrodesis procedures seems to be driven by a combination of radiological and clinical considerations. In a survey inquiring foot and ankle surgeons about the need for bone graft in arthrodesis procedures, the top 3 clinical factors motivating the use of bone graft were the presence of nonunion or previous history of nonunion, followed by smoking and concomitant medications that are known to impede bone healing.[73] On the other hand, evidence of nonunion, avascular necrosis, and incongruous bone apposition with bone gap were the main radiological factors influencing surgeons' decision on using a bone graft. Although bone grafting in high-risk patients and nonunion revision surgeries is common, the evidence supporting it is unclear or insufficient. As a successful union depends on multiple factors (mechanical stability, comorbidities, surgical technic, and complexity) it is extremely difficult to obtain non-union rates based purely on the use of bone graft. The review by Lareau and colleagues is perhaps the most extensive analysis made up today.[74] They performed a logistic regression analysis of 159 studies in the foot and ankle literature comparing the use of autograft, allograft, and no bone graft for foot and ankle arthrodesis. Among other results, they demonstrated a trend toward higher union rates with autograft and cancellous allograft relative to no graft. Although no differences were statistically significant, the addition of bone graft approximately halved the nonunion rate. They conclude that considering the frequency, expense, functional impairment, and comorbidity of failed arthrodesis, this difference could be viewed as clinically substantial.

Overall, insufficient evidence supports the routine use of bone autograft or suitable alternatives to enhance fusion in ankle and hindfoot arthrodesis. Nevertheless, using bone grafts in more complex cases, high-risk patients, nonunion revision surgeries, and the filling-in of bone voids in the arthrodesis site to improve bone apposition should be considered to improve results and union rates, as the benefits of their use outweigh the drawbacks.

Autologous bone graft: Anterior iliac crest or proximal tibia?
Despite the dramatic advances in the orthobiological industry during the past decades, the autologous bone graft is still the gold standard for improving healing in arthrodesis and nonunion revision surgeries. This is mainly owing to its naturally osteoconductive, osteoinductive, and osteogenic characteristics.[74] Furthermore, it negates the potential risk of immunologic and infectious complications associated with the use of allograft.[75]

Traditionally, autologous bone is harvested from the anterior iliac crest. Because it can provide large quantities of cancellous and cortical bone, the iliac crest is ideal in situations whereby structural support may be required, such as ankle arthrodesis with more significant bone defects and subtalar distraction arthrodesis. Additionally, the iliac crest bone possesses higher marrow content, resulting in greater osteogenic potential compared with other anatomic sites.[76] For these reasons, the iliac crest is considered the gold standard site for bone harvesting. However, high incidence (20%–40%) of potential complications and several drawbacks have been associated with bone harvesting at the iliac crest, including hematoma, infection, chronic pain, nerve injury, fracture, and hypertrophic scar.[76] As an alternative, other sites for bone harvesting have gained increased popularity, namely the calcaneus and proximal and distal tibia.[75] In addition to being close to the operative site, which facilitates tourniquet and draping placement, a significant amount of bone graft can be obtained. On average, 30 cc can be harvested from the proximal tibia, which is suitable for most foot and ankle procedures.[77] The incidence of complications related to proximal tibial bone grafting has been reported as extremely low (1.3%) and include tibial tubercle fracture, hematoma, and superficial infection.[78]

Although the iliac crest presents superior histologic features, there is no evidence supporting the use over other sites in terms of union rates for foot and ankle surgery. However, proximal tibial bone harvesting can be a valid alternative because of its simplicity and low incidence of associated complications.

Orthobiologics

Orthobiologics are biologically active substances used therapeutically for their positive effects on healing skeletal and soft-tissue injuries. Several orthobiologics products are currently available to the foot and ankle surgeon, including bone allografts, bone substitutes, and growth factors. To better elucidate their role in foot and ankle arthrodesis, these different types of orthobiologics can be grouped according to their primary function: (1) to provide structural support; (2) to address bone defects; (3) as augmentation in joint fusion surgeries.

Structural support is often required in complex hindfoot reconstruction and arthrodesis procedures, such as subtalar distraction and ankle arthrodesis with substantial bone defects. Of the orthobiologics, the cortical and cortico-cancellous bone allografts are frequently used to provide structural support as they are more rigid and resistant to loading forces.[79] Bone allografts obviate the inherent donor site problems of autogenous bone grafts but are beset by issues with graft rejection, low osteogenic and osteoinductive properties, and slower graft incorporation, particularly in areas whereby the blood supply is comparatively tenuous. Nonetheless, there seems to be no significant difference in well-vascularized bone sites when comparing incorporation and complication rates of allografts versus autogenous grafts.[79]

Bone defects whereby no physical support is needed can be addressed with different orthobiologics such as cancellous bone allograft, demineralized bone matrix (DBM), and bone graft substitutes.[80] Cancellous bone graft is often used but has the issues inherent to all allografts. DBM is a form of allograft prepared by acid extraction, so it retains bone morphogenetic proteins (BMP) and bone collagens. Therefore, DBM has improved osteoinductive capacity compared with traditional allograft, and available evidence seems to support the use of DBM in ankle and hindfoot joint fusion procedures.[79,80] However, the data are essentially retrospective with small samples and typically involves short-term follow-up. As an alternative to allografts and associated complications, synthetic bone graft substitutes, such as calcium phosphate and calcium sulfate, can be implanted to treat bone defects.[79] The clinical utility of these materials lies in their 3D porous structure that provides an osteoconductive scaffold, which enhances the adhesion and proliferation of osteoprogenitor cells, and correspondingly promotes the growth of new bone.[79] They are commonly used as an adjunct to bone reconstruction in trauma surgery, and their use in foot and ankle arthrodesis surgery seems more uncommon.

The use of augmentation products to improve fusion in foot and ankle arthrodesis has been gaining popularity as their use in foot and ankle procedures has been approved in different countries worldwide.[80] Platelet-derived growth factor (PDGF) and platelet-rich plasma (PRP) are perhaps the products more commonly used and with the more available evidence.[81] PDGF is a polypeptide growth factor released by platelets and macrophages in the injury site and plays a role in embryogenesis, angiogenesis, and osteogenesis.[80] The use of rhPDGF in foot and ankle arthrodesis procedures has shown significant equivalent clinical outcomes in bone fusion performance compared with the autologous bone graft.[82] Moreover, compared with autologous bone graft, the use of rhPDGF was associated with fewer adverse events such as chronic graft site pain.

The rationale for using PRP lies in the anabolic and immune-modulatory properties of platelet concentrates. When activated, platelets release a group of biologically active proteins, such as growth factors and cytokines, crucial for bone, cartilage, and soft-tissue healing.[83] In the foot and ankle, PRP is frequently used in cartilage and soft tissues lesions, and its safety has been demonstrated.[84] However, the evidence supporting PRP to enhance bone healing seems to be scarce and quite contradictory. The use of PRP augmentation has been associated with higher fusion rates and reduced time to fusion in some studies, while others have shown no differences.[85,86] Regardless of this disparity, it seems to be unanimous that PRP augmentation is a safe method to deliver active biological factors to the fusion site, with few risks associated.

Postoperative Factors

Pain medications

The impact of nonsteroid antiinflammatory (NSAID) medications on bone healing is a topic of intense discussion. It is thought that the use of NSAID medication in postoperative pain management can affect the typical inflammatory cascade needed for new bone formation, thus, increasing the risk of developing a nonunion.[87] Most of the available data assessing the effects of NSAID in bone healing involves patients with bone fractures, and little is known about the influence of these medications in foot and ankle arthrodesis outcomes. A recent meta-analyis of 16 studies with a total of 15,242 bones included investigated whether the use of NSAIDs increased the risk of delayed and nonunion in the setting of fracture, osteotomy, or fusion procedure.[88] Their results revealed that the effect of NSAIDs on delayed or nonunion is strongly related to patients' age. There was an increased risk of delayed or nonunion with NSAID exposure (OR 2.07) in the adult population, suggesting that this medication can be safely administered in pediatric patients without compromising bone healing. In addition, this study found that a low dose or short postoperative exposure to NSAIDs did not substantially increase the risk of delayed or nonunion. NSAIDs seem to have dose-dependent and duration-dependent effects on fusion rates. However, short-term (<2 weeks) postoperative use seems to have no effect on nonunion rates.[89]

Because there are multiple confounding factors in the bone healing process, the actual role of these medications as a non-union risk factor is still not fully determined. Nevertheless, based on current evidence, pain management with NSAIDs should be limited to a short period and avoided in high-risk patients after an arthrodesis procedure.

Early vs. delayed weight-bearing

Non-weight-bearing has been traditionally recommended after foot and ankle arthrodesis as early weight-bearing and repetitive loading may increase micromotion at the fusion site, increasing the risk of nonunion. On the other hand, it has been demonstrated that bone healing is enhanced by micromovements of bone fragments, as bone remodeling and mass density are directly linked with direct load-bearing.[90] In addition, non–weight-bearing after lower extremity surgeries is associated with increased bone demineralization, muscle atrophy, and thromboembolic events.[91,92] For these reasons, historical non–weight-bearing protocols have been questioned

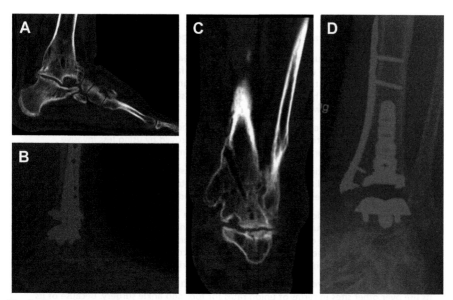

Fig. 3. Pre and postoperative imaging of a 59-year-old female patient presenting with symptomatic end-stage subtalar osteoarthritis 4 years after an ankle fusion for ankle osteoarthritis. For this patient, a take-down fusion and conversion to total ankle arthroplasty (Inbone, Wright medical) was performed. (*A*) Preoperative ankle CT sagittal view showing ankle fusion with subtalar osteoarthritis. (*B*) Postoperative weight-bearing lateral ankle radiograph. (*C*) Preoperative ankle CT coronal view showing ankle fusion with subtalar osteoarthritis. (*D*) Postoperative weight-bearing AP ankle radiograph 6 months after total ankle conversion with a medial malleolus plate reinforcement.

by an increasing number of studies being conducted in this field and recent randomized controlled trials comparing short-term outcomes of early versus delayed weight-bearing after ankle fracture fixation has shown that early weight-bearing is associated with better general health status, better function, earlier return to work, and sport without increased postoperative complications.[93–95] Although short-term outcomes are pretty promising, these studies did not investigate the influence of early weight-bearing in time-to-union and nonunion rates.

Early weight-bearing after arthrodesis surgery in the foot and ankle remains poorly researched without high-level evidence studies. A recent systematic review aiming to compare outcomes between early and delayed weight-bearing protocols after ankle arthrodesis was conducted by Potter and colleagues in 2019.[96] A total of 2426 ankles were included and divided into 4 groups according to the duration of the postoperative non–weight-bearing period: zero to 1 week (group A), 2 to 3 weeks (group B), 4 to 5 weeks (group C), or 6 weeks or more (group D). Mean union rates for groups A to D were 93.2%, 95.5%, 93.0%, and 93.0%, respectively. No clear trend was found between groups when comparing the time required to achieve union. Mean time to union was 10.4 weeks, 14.5 weeks, 12.4 weeks, and 14.4 weeks for groups A to D, respectively. The shortest time to union was found in the group with early weight-bearing supporting the hypothesis that early weight-bearing may promote faster union.

Regarding complication rates, the mean was 22.3%, 23.0%, 27.1%, and 28.7% for groups A to D, respectively. Although similar rates were generally found between groups, early weight-bearing was associated with a slightly lower incidence of

---

Box 1
Main clinic care points relevant to improve outcomes of foot and ankle arthrodesis procedures

- There is fair evidence supporting smoking and diabetes as a risk factor for nonunion following foot and ankle arthrodesis for preoperative factors. However, through smoking cessation and good diabetic control before the procedure, surgeons may improve outcomes. Moreover, screening and hypovitaminosis D treatment supplementation is recommended as the benefits seem to outweigh the risks.

- When technically feasible, less invasive techniques should be the first choice as patient outcomes and postoperative complications can be improved by using less invasive techniques, even in the presence of more severe deformities.

- Regarding joint preparation, surgeons should use twist drills rather than Kirschner wires, prefer drill bits of small diameter, decrease the time interval between passes, drilling at more perpendicular angles, apply regular irrigation and bone debris evacuation.

- There is insufficient evidence supporting the routine use of bone autograft or suitable alternatives to enhance fusion in primary ankle and hindfoot arthrodesis. Nevertheless, using bone grafts in more complex cases, high-risk patients, nonunion revision surgeries, and filling in bone voids at the arthrodesis site, should be considered to improve results and union rates, as the benefits of their use outweigh the risks.

- Although the iliac crest presents superior histologic features, there is no evidence supporting its use over other sites in terms of union rates for foot and ankle surgery. Because of its simplicity and low incidence of associated complications, proximal tibial bone harvesting can be a valid alternative.

- The use of orthobiologics, namely rhPDGF, in foot and ankle arthrodesis procedures has shown equivalent clinical outcomes and bone fusion performance compared with autologous bone graft. Moreover, the use of orthobiologics may obviate adverse events and morbidity related to autologous bone graft harvesting.

- Based on current evidence, pain management with NSAIDs should be limited to a short period (<2 weeks) and avoided in high-risk patients after an arthrodesis procedure.

- Although evidence is quite limited, early postoperative weight-bearing has shown to be beneficial, and it does not seem to increase postoperative complications. Therefore, it seems reasonable to start weight-bearing at an early phase when the arthrodesis is performed in loading joints with low shear forces.

- The incidence of surrounding joint osteoarthritis after foot and ankle fusion seems to increase progressively with time. Owing to its progression and high probability of being symptomatic, patients must be informed consequently, as they may require additional joint fusions, resulting in further loss of ankle/foot motion.

- In patients with symptomatic adjacent joint OA and unsatisfactory results after an ankle arthrodesis, conversion to total ankle arthroplasty (TAA) has become a potential option in managing these complex and challenging situations.

---

complications overall. The authors conclude that outcomes following ankle arthrodesis seem to be similar regardless of the duration of postoperative non–weight-bearing period, although, the existing literature is insufficient to make definitive conclusions.

Early weight-bearing versus delayed weight-bearing after midfoot joint arthrodesis has also been investigated. In a comparative, multicenter retrospective study involving 367 patients undergoing modified Lapidus arthrodesis with various fixation constructs, early weight-bearing did not increase the risk of nonunion than delayed weight-bearing.[97] These results support previous findings, suggesting that non–weight-bearing after tarsometatarsal arthrodesis may not be necessary.[98,99] Regarding arthrodesis of the first metatarsophalangeal, similar conclusions can be made as evidence shows no differences in nonunion rates with early weight-bearing.[63,100]

Overall, the heterogenicity of the available studies and paucity of level I-II studies do not allow definite conclusions and correctly recommend early over delayed weight-bearing in foot and ankle arthrodesis. However, there is a general trend to abandon long, non–weight-bearing periods as current evidence favors early weight-bearing. Early postoperative weight-bearing has shown to be beneficial, and it does not seem to increase postoperative complications. It is possible that although early weight-bearing may enhance compression and coaptation in some joints (eg, ankle and subtalar), a similar protocol in other joints (eg, talonavicular) may increase shear under physiologic loads and compromise fusion site stability. Therefore, given patients' satisfaction with early weight-bearing and low compliance to long periods of non–weight-bearing, it seems reasonable to start weight-bearing at an early phase when the arthrodesis is performed in loading joints with low shear forces.

FUTURE OF SURROUNDING JOINTS

Osteoarthritis in surrounding joints is a major concern after foot and ankle arthrodesis procedures. It has been demonstrated that fusion of the ankle joint results in decreased eversion/inversion and internal/external rotation of the subtalar joint, which increases the mechanical stress of the subtalar joint during walking.[101] Consequently, this joint overloading can lead to progressive joint degeneration, which results in later osteoarthritis. It seems that the overloading of surrounding joints starts a few months following the arthrodesis procedure, as demonstrated in a recent study whereby postoperative SPECT-CT performed in patients undergoing ankle arthrodesis showed significantly increased activity in surrounding joints 6 months after surgery.[102] In addition, the incidence of surrounding joint osteoarthritis after ankle fusion seems to increase progressively with time. Coester and colleagues reported that secondary subtalar OA developed or progressed in 33% of patients at 9 years and 90% at 22 years after the primary ankle fusion.[103] Regarding talonavicular OA, 37% of patients developed or progressed OA at 9 years and 55% at 22 years after the ankle fusion. One could say that this degenerative process is bidirectional, as ankle OA seems to develop or progress in 55% of patients 15 years after a triple hindfoot arthrodesis.[104] Similar overloading mechanisms seem to explain the 30% midterm incidence of adjacent joint OA after isolated talonavicular arthrodesis.[105]

Overall, adjacent joint OA after arthrodesis procedures is frequently encountered in the foot and ankle. Owing to its progression and high probability of being symptomatic, patients must be informed consequently, as they may require additional joint fusions, resulting in further loss of ankle/foot motion. For instance, a young patient who undergoes ankle arthrodesis is likely to develop hindfoot osteoarthritis during the next 20 years, which may lead to additional hindfoot fusion surgery.[103,106,107] In this scenario, the risk of nonunion in the setting of previous ipsilateral ankle/hindfoot fusion is substantially higher as 40%.[108] Additionally, patients undergoing multiple foot and ankle fusions often have difficulties performing daily-basis activities such as climbing stairs, getting out of a chair, walking on uneven surfaces, and running.[109] Thus, patient satisfaction and disability level seem to decline with time.[103]

In patients with symptomatic adjacent joint OA and unsatisfactory results after an ankle arthrodesis, conversion to total ankle arthroplasty (TAA) has become a potential option in managing these complex and challenging situations. As improved instrumentation and more significant experience with TAA have facilitated this procedure, the number of reports involving patients undergoing take-down fusion and conversion to TAA has been increasing during the last decade. A recent systematic review involving 172 patients submitted to this procedure with a mean follow-up of 62.8 months, reported substantial pain (mean preoperative VAS 7.8 vs 2.5 postoperatively) and ankle function improvement (mean preoperative AOFAS score 32 vs 72.4 postoperatively) after surgery.[110] However, long-term outcomes have not been reported. An example of pre and postoperative imaging of a take-down ankle fusion and conversion to TAA is illustrated in **Fig. 3**.

Take-down fusion is a complex procedure and should be performed by surgeons with extensive experience in total ankle arthroplasty procedures. Although the evidence is scarce, conversion of ankle arthrodesis to total ankle replacement seems to be a viable option to improve patient outcomes and prevent extensive hindfoot arthrodesis.

SUMMARY

Determining who is at risk of developing complications is essential to reduce the nonunion rates and improve patient outcomes after foot and ankle arthrodesis. However, a successful joint fusion depends on a complex relationship of several factors, such as patient-related factors, intraoperative, and postoperative factors. Therefore, research performed in this field often has inherent methodological limitations, which difficults to provide a definitive conclusion. Based on the current evidence, several conclusions can be drawn and are summarized in **Box 1**.

CLINICS CARE POINTS

- There is fair evidence supporting smoking and diabetes as a risk factor for non-union following foot and ankle arthrodesis for preoperative factors.
- Less invasive techniques should be the first choice as patient outcomes and postoperative complications can be improved.
- There is insufficient evidence supporting the routine use of bone autograft or suitable alternatives to enhance fusion in primary ankle and hindfoot arthrodesis.
- Although the iliac crest presents superior histological features, there is no evidence supporting its use over other sites in terms of union rates for foot and ankle surgery.
- The use of orthobiologics, namely rhPDGF, in foot and ankle arthrodesis procedures has shown equivalent clinical outcomes and bone fusion performance compared to autologous bone graft.
- Although evidence is quite limited, early postoperative weight-bearing has shown to be beneficial, and it does not seem to increase postoperative complications.
- Based on current evidence, pain management with NSAIDs should be limited to a short period (<2 weeks) and avoided in high-risk patients after an arthrodesis procedure.

DISCLOSURE

The authors have nothing to disclose.

REFERENCES

1. O'Connor KM, Johnson JE, McCormick JJ, et al. Clinical and operative factors related to successful revision arthrodesis in the foot and ankle. Foot Ankle Int 2016;37(8):809–15.

2. Thevendran G, Wang C, Pinney SJ, et al. Nonunion Risk Assessment in Foot and Ankle Surgery: Proposing a Predictive Risk Assessment Model. Foot Ankle Int 2015;36(8):901–7.
3. Ma S, Jin D. Isolated Talonavicular Arthrodesis. Foot Ankle Int 2016;37(8):905–8.
4. Gougoulias N, Lampridis V. Midfoot arthrodesis. Foot Ankle Surg 2016;22(1): 17–25.
5. Brown CW, Orme TJ, Richardson HD. The rate of pseudarthrosis (surgical nonunion) in patients who are smokers and patients who are nonsmokers: a comparison study. Spine (Phila Pa 1976) 1986;11(9):942–3.
6. Cobb TK, Gabrielsen TA, Campbell DC 2nd, et al. Cigarette smoking and nonunion after ankle arthrodesis. Foot Ankle Int 1994;15(2):64–7.
7. Thevendran G, Shah K, Pinney SJ, et al. Perceived risk factors for nonunion following foot and ankle arthrodesis. J Orthop Surg 2017;25(1). 230949901769270.
8. Giannoudis PV, Einhorn TA, Marsh D. Fracture healing: a harmony of optimal biology and optimal fixation? Injury 2007;38(Suppl 4):S1–2.
9. Beahrs TR, Reagan J, Bettin CC, et al. Smoking Effects in Foot and Ankle Surgery: An Evidence-Based Review. Foot Ankle Int 2019;40(10):1226–32.
10. Al-Bashaireh AM, Haddad LG, Weaver M, et al. The Effect of Tobacco Smoking on Musculoskeletal Health: A Systematic Review. J Environ Public Health 2018; 2018:4184190.
11. Heyes G, Weigelt L, Molloy A, et al. The influence of smoking on foot and ankle surgery: a review of the literature. Foot (Edinb). 2021;46:101735.
12. Thevendran G, Younger A, Pinney S. Current concepts review: risk factors for nonunions in foot and ankle arthrodeses. Foot Ankle Int 2012;33(11):1031–40.
13. Shipton D, Tappin DM, Vadiveloo T, et al. Reliability of self reported smoking status by pregnant women for estimating smoking prevalence: a retrospective, cross sectional study. Bmj 2009;339:b4347.
14. Etzel RA. A review of the use of saliva cotinine as a marker of tobacco smoke exposure. Prev Med 1990;19(2):190–7.
15. Lee JJ, Patel R, Biermann JS, et al. The musculoskeletal effects of cigarette smoking. J Bone Joint Surg Am 2013;95(9):850–9.
16. Mills E, Eyawo O, Lockhart I, et al. Smoking cessation reduces postoperative complications: a systematic review and meta-analysis. Am J Med 2011; 124(2):144–54.e148.
17. Sorensen LT, Karlsmark T, Gottrup F. Abstinence from smoking reduces incisional wound infection: a randomized controlled trial. Ann Surg 2003;238(1):1–5.
18. Childs BR, Nahm NJ, Dolenc AJ, et al. Obesity Is Associated With More Complications and Longer Hospital Stays After Orthopaedic Trauma. J Orthop Trauma 2015;29(11):504–9.
19. Benedick A, Audet MA, Vallier HA. The effect of obesity on post-operative complications and functional outcomes after surgical treatment of torsional ankle fracture: A matched cohort study. Injury 2020;51(8):1893–8.
20. Thorud JC, Mortensen S, Thorud JL, et al. Effect of Obesity on Bone Healing After Foot and Ankle Long Bone Fractures. J Foot Ankle Surg 2017;56(2):258–62.
21. Cardoso DV, Paccaud J, Dubois-Ferrière V, et al. The effect of BMI on long-term outcomes after operatively treated ankle fractures: a study with up to 16 years of follow-up. BMC Musculoskelet Disord 2022;23(1):317.
22. Siboni R, Beaufils P, Boisrenoult P, et al. Opening-wedge high tibial osteotomy without bone grafting in severe varus osteoarthritic knee. Rate and risk factors of non-union in 41 cases. Orthop Traumatol Surg Res 2018;104(4):473–6.

23. Liska F, Haller B, Voss A, et al. Smoking and obesity influence the risk of nonunion in lateral opening wedge, closing wedge and torsional distal femoral osteotomies. Knee Surg Sports Traumatol Arthrosc 2018;26(9):2551–7.

24. Elamir Y, Gianakos AL, Lane JM, et al. The Effects of Diabetes and Diabetic Medications on Bone Health. J Orthop Trauma 2020;34(3):e102–8.

25. Gortler H, Rusyn J, Godbout C, et al. Diabetes and Healing Outcomes in Lower Extremity Fractures: A Systematic Review. Injury 2018;49(2):177–83.

26. Falanga V. Wound healing and its impairment in the diabetic foot. Lancet 2005; 366(9498):1736–43.

27. Myers TG, Lowery NJ, Frykberg RG, et al. Ankle and hindfoot fusions: comparison of outcomes in patients with and without diabetes. Foot Ankle Int 2012; 33(1):20–8.

28. Boulton AJ, Vileikyte L, Ragnarson-Tennvall G, et al. The global burden of diabetic foot disease. Lancet 2005;366(9498):1719–24.

29. Shibuya N, Humphers JM, Fluhman BL, et al. Factors associated with nonunion, delayed union, and malunion in foot and ankle surgery in diabetic patients. J Foot Ankle Surg 2013;52(2):207–11.

30. Fischer V, Haffner-Luntzer M, Amling M, et al. Calcium and vitamin D in bone fracture healing and post-traumatic bone turnover. Eur Cell Mater 2018;35: 365–85.

31. Aujla RS, Allen PE, Ribbans WJ. Vitamin D levels in 577 consecutive elective foot & ankle surgery patients. Foot Ankle Surg 2019;25(3):310–5.

32. Smith JT, Halim K, Palms DA, et al. Prevalence of vitamin D deficiency in patients with foot and ankle injuries. Foot Ankle Int 2014;35(1):8–13.

33. Moore KR, Howell MA, Saltrick KR, et al. Risk Factors Associated With Nonunion After Elective Foot and Ankle Reconstruction: A Case-Control Study. J Foot Ankle Surg 2017;56(3):457–62.

34. Doetsch AM, Faber J, Lynnerup N, et al. The effect of calcium and vitamin D3 supplementation on the healing of the proximal humerus fracture: a randomized placebo-controlled study. Calcif Tissue Int 2004;75(3):183–8.

35. Pountos I, Georgouli T, Blokhuis TJ, et al. Pharmacological agents and impairment of fracture healing: what is the evidence? Injury 2008;39(4):384–94.

36. Gaston MS, Simpson AH. Inhibition of fracture healing. J Bone Joint Surg Br 2007;89(12):1553–60.

37. Sawin PD, Dickman CA, Crawford NR, et al. The effects of dexamethasone on bone fusion in an experimental model of posterolateral lumbar spinal arthrodesis. J Neurosurg 2001;94(1 Suppl):76–81.

38. Satoh K, Mark H, Zachrisson P, et al. Effect of methotrexate on fracture healing. Fukushima J Med Sci. 2011;57(1):11-18.

39. Pountos I, Giannoudis PV. Effect of methotrexate on bone and wound healing. Expert Opin Drug Saf. 2017;16(5):535-545.

40. Hazan EJ, Hornicek FJ, Tomford W, et al. The effect of adjuvant chemotherapy on osteoarticular allografts. Clin Orthop Relat Res 2001;385:176–81.

41. Huddleston PM, Steckelberg JM, Hanssen AD, et al. Ciprofloxacin inhibition of experimental fracture healing. J Bone Joint Surg Am 2000;82(2):161–73.

42. Michels F, Guillo S, De Lavigne C, et al. The arthroscopic Lapidus procedure. Foot Ankle Surg 2011;17(1):25–8.

43. Lui TH, Chan KB, Ng S. Arthroscopic Lapidus arthrodesis. Arthroscopy 2005; 21(12):1516.

44. Vernois J, Redfern D. Lapidus, a Percutaneous Approach. Foot Ankle Clin 2020; 25(3):407–12.

45. Mok TN, He Q, Panneerselavam S, et al. Open versus arthroscopic ankle arthrodesis: a systematic review and meta-analysis. J Orthop Surg Res 2020; 15(1):187.
46. Townshend D, Di Silvestro M, Krause F, et al. Arthroscopic versus open ankle arthrodesis: a multicenter comparative case series. J bone Jt Surg Am volume 2013;95(2):98–102.
47. Quayle J, Shafafy R, Khan MA, et al. Arthroscopic versus open ankle arthrodesis. Foot Ankle Surg 2018;24(2):137–42.
48. Woo BJ, Lai MC, Ng S, et al. Clinical outcomes comparing arthroscopic vs open ankle arthrodesis. Foot Ankle Surg 2020;26(5):530–4.
49. Baumbach SF, Massen FK, Hörterer S, et al. Comparison of arthroscopic to open tibiotalocalcaneal arthrodesis in high-risk patients. Foot Ankle Surg 2019;25(6):804–11.
50. Dannawi Z, Nawabi DH, Patel A, et al. Arthroscopic ankle arthrodesis: are results reproducible irrespective of pre-operative deformity? Foot Ankle Surg 2011;17(4):294–9.
51. Yang TC, Tzeng YH, Wang CS, et al. Arthroscopic Ankle Arthrodesis Provides Similarly Satisfactory Surgical Outcomes in Ankles With Severe Deformity Compared With Mild Deformity in Elderly Patients. Arthroscopy 2020;36(10): 2738–47.
52. Issac RT, Thomson LE, Khan K, et al. Do degree of coronal plane deformity and patient related factors affect union and outcome of Arthroscopic versus Open Ankle Arthrodesis? Foot Ankle Surg 2021;28(5):635–41.
53. Rungprai C, Jaroenarpornwatana A, Chaiprom N, et al. Outcomes and Complications of Open vs Posterior Arthroscopic Subtalar Arthrodesis: A Prospective Randomized Controlled Multicenter Study[Formula: see text]. Foot Ankle Int 2021;42(11):1371–83.
54. Rungprai C, Phisitkul P, Femino JE, et al. Outcomes and Complications After Open Versus Posterior Arthroscopic Subtalar Arthrodesis in 121 Patients. J Bone Joint Surg Am 2016;98(8):636–46.
55. ross KA, Seaworth CM, Smyth NA, Ling JS, Sayres SC, Kennedy JG. Talonavicular arthroscopy for osteochondral lesions: technique and case series. *Foot Ankle Int.* 2014;35(9):909-915.56.
56. Jagodzinski NA, Parsons AM, Parsons SW. Arthroscopic triple and modified double hindfoot arthrodesis. *Foot Ankle Surg.* 2015;21(2):97-102.57.
57. Vieira Cardoso D, Veljkovic A, Wing K, Penner M, Gagne O, Younger A. Cohort Comparison of Radiographic Correction and Complications Between Minimal Invasive and Open Lapidus Procedures for Hallux Valgus. *Foot Ankle Int.* 2022:10711007221112088
58. Hefti FL, Baumann JU, Morscher EW. Ankle joint fusion – determination of optimal position by gait analysis. Arch Orthop Trauma Surg (1978 1980;96(3): 187–95.
59. Muir DC, Amendola A, Saltzman CL. Long-term outcome of ankle arthrodesis. Foot Ankle Clin 2002;7(4):703–8.
60. Miniaci-Coxhead SL, Weisenthal B, Ketz JP, et al. Incidence and Radiographic Predictors of Valgus Tibiotalar Tilt After Hindfoot Fusion. Foot Ankle Int 2017; 38(5):519–25.
61. De Cesar Netto C, Ahrenholz S, Iehl C, et al. Lapicotton technique in the treatment of progressive collapsing foot deformity. J Foot Ankle 2020;14(3):301–8.
62. Augustin G, Davila S, Mihoci K, et al. Thermal osteonecrosis and bone drilling parameters revisited. Arch Orthop Trauma Surg 2008;128(1):71–7.

63. Korim MT, Mahadevan D, Ghosh A, et al. Effect of joint pathology, surface preparation and fixation methods on union frequency after first metatarsophalangeal joint arthrodesis: A systematic review of the English literature. Foot Ankle Surg 2017;23(3):189–94.

64. Schmid T, Krause F. The modified Lapidus fusion. Foot Ankle Clin 2014;19(2): 223–33.

65. Boffeli TJ, Hyllengren SB. Can We Abandon Saw Wedge Resection in Lapidus Fusion? A Comparative Study of Joint Preparation Techniques Regarding Correction of Deformity, Union Rate, and Preservation of First Ray Length. J Foot Ankle Surg 2019;58(6):1118–24.

66. Tai BL, Palmisano AC, Belmont B, Irwin TA, Holmes J, Shih AJ. Numerical evaluation of sequential bone drilling strategies based on thermal damage. Med Eng Phys. 2015;37(9):855-861.67.

67. Lee J, Chavez CL, Park J. Parameters affecting mechanical and thermal responses in bone drilling: A review. J Biomech. 2018;71:4-21.

68. Meeson R, Moazen M, Sanghani-Kerai A, et al. The influence of gap size on the development of fracture union with a micro external fixator. J Mech Behav Biomed Mater 2019;99:161–8.

69. Harrison LJ, Cunningham JL, Strömberg L, et al. Controlled Induction of a Pseudarthrosis: A Study Using a Rodent Model. J Orthop Trauma 2003;17(1):11–21.

70. DiGiovanni CW, Lin SS, Daniels TR, et al. The Importance of Sufficient Graft Material in Achieving Foot or Ankle Fusion. J Bone Joint Surg Am 2016;98(15): 1260–7.

71. Heifner JJ, Monir JG, Reb CW. Impact of Bone Graft on Fusion Rates in Primary Open Ankle Arthrodesis Fixated With Cannulated Screws: A Systematic Review. J Foot Ankle Surg 2021;60(4):802–6.

72. Buda M, Hagemeijer NC, Kink S, et al. Effect of Fixation Type and Bone Graft on Tarsometatarsal Fusion. Foot Ankle Int 2018;39(12):1394–402.

73. Baumhauer JF, Pinzur MS, Daniels TR, et al. Survey on the need for bone graft in foot and ankle fusion surgery. Foot Ankle Int 2013;34(12):1629–33.

74. Lareau CR, Deren ME, Fantry A, et al. Does autogenous bone graft work? A logistic regression analysis of data from 159 papers in the foot and ankle literature. Foot Ankle Surg 2015;21(3):150–9.

75. Winson IG, Higgs A. The use of proximal and distal tibial bone graft in foot and ankle procedures. Foot Ankle Clin 2010;15(4):553–8.

76. Dimitriou R, Mataliotakis GI, Angoules AG, et al. Complications following autologous bone graft harvesting from the iliac crest and using the RIA: a systematic review. Injury 2011;42(Suppl 2):S3–15.

77. Geideman W, Early JS, Brodsky J. Clinical results of harvesting autogenous cancellous graft from the ipsilateral proximal tibia for use in foot and ankle surgery. Foot Ankle Int 2004;25(7):451–5.

78. O'Keeffe RM Jr, Riemer BL, Butterfield SL. Harvesting of autogenous cancellous bone graft from the proximal tibial metaphysis. A review of 230 cases. J Orthop Trauma 1991;5(4):469–74.

79. Wee J, Thevendran G. The role of orthobiologics in foot and ankle surgery: Allogenic bone grafts and bone graft substitutes. EFORT Open Rev 2017;2(6): 272–80.

80. Yeoh JC, Taylor BA. Osseous Healing in Foot and Ankle Surgery with Autograft, Allograft, and Other Orthobiologics. Orthop Clin North Am 2017;48(3):359–69.

81. Lin SS, Yeranosian MG. The Role of Orthobiologics in Fracture Healing and Arthrodesis. Foot Ankle Clin 2016;21(4):727–37.

82. Daniels TR, Younger AS, Penner MJ, et al. Prospective Randomized Controlled Trial of Hindfoot and Ankle Fusions Treated With rhPDGF-BB in Combination With a β-TCP-Collagen Matrix. Foot Ankle Int 2015;36(7):739–48.
83. Bibbo C, Hatfield PS. Platelet-rich plasma concentrate to augment bone fusion. Foot Ankle Clin 2010;15(4):641–9.
84. Vieira Cardoso D, Ruffieux E, Valisena S, et al. [Management of ankle osteoarthritis in the young adult]. Rev Med Suisse 2021;17(763):2173–9.
85. Coetzee JC, Pomeroy GC, Watts JD, et al. The use of autologous concentrated growth factors to promote syndesmosis fusion in the Agility total ankle replacement. A preliminary study. Foot Ankle Int 2005;26(10):840–6.
86. Bibbo C, Bono CM, Lin SS. Union rates using autologous platelet concentrate alone and with bone graft in high-risk foot and ankle surgery patients. J Surg Orthop Adv 2005;14(1):17–22.
87. Richards CJ, Graf KW Jr, Mashru RP. The Effect of Opioids, Alcohol, and Nonsteroidal Anti-inflammatory Drugs on Fracture Union. Orthop Clin North Am 2017;48(4):433–43.
88. Wheatley BM, Nappo KE, Christensen DL, et al. Effect of NSAIDs on Bone Healing Rates: A Meta-analysis. J Am Acad Orthop Surg 2019;27(7):e330–6.
89. Sivaganesan A, Chotai S, White-Dzuro G, et al. The effect of NSAIDs on spinal fusion: a cross-disciplinary review of biochemical, animal, and human studies. Eur Spine J 2017;26(11):2719–28.
90. Bailón-Plaza A, van der Meulen MC. Beneficial effects of moderate, early loading and adverse effects of delayed or excessive loading on bone healing. J Biomech 2003;36(8):1069–77.
91. Ito M, Matsumoto T, Enomoto H, et al. Effect of nonweight bearing on tibial bone density measured by QCT in patients with hip surgery. J Bone Miner Metab 1999;17(1):45–50.
92. de Boer MD, Seynnes OR, di Prampero PE, et al. Effect of 5 weeks horizontal bed rest on human muscle thickness and architecture of weight bearing and non-weight bearing muscles. Eur J Appl Physiol 2008;104(2):401–7.
93. Dehghan N, McKee MD, Jenkinson RJ, et al. Early Weightbearing and Range of Motion Versus Non-Weightbearing and Immobilization After Open Reduction and Internal Fixation of Unstable Ankle Fractures: A Randomized Controlled Trial. J Orthop Trauma 2016;30(7):345–52.
94. Smeeing DPJ, Houwert RM, Briet JP, et al. Weight-bearing or non-weight-bearing after surgical treatment of ankle fractures: a multicenter randomized controlled trial. Eur J Trauma Emerg Surg 2020;46(1):121–30.
95. Schubert J, Lambers KTA, Kimber C, et al. Effect on Overall Health Status With Weightbearing at 2 Weeks vs 6 Weeks After Open Reduction and Internal Fixation of Ankle Fractures. Foot Ankle Int 2020;41(6):658–65.
96. Potter MJ, Freeman R. Postoperative weightbearing following ankle arthrodesis: a systematic review. Bone Joint J 2019;101-b(10):1256–62.
97. Prissel MA, Hyer CF, Grambart ST, et al. A Multicenter, Retrospective Study of Early Weightbearing for Modified Lapidus Arthrodesis. J Foot Ankle Surg 2016;55(2):226–9.
98. King CM, Richey J, Patel S, et al. Modified lapidus arthrodesis with crossed screw fixation: early weightbearing in 136 patients. J Foot Ankle Surg 2015; 54(1):69–75.
99. Ray JJ, Koay J, Dayton PD, et al. Multicenter Early Radiographic Outcomes of Triplanar Tarsometatarsal Arthrodesis With Early Weightbearing. Foot Ankle Int 2019;40(8):955–60.

100. Crowell A, Van JC, Meyr AJ. Early Weight-Bearing After Arthrodesis of the First Metatarsal-Phalangeal Joint: A Systematic Review of the Incidence of Non-Union. J Foot Ankle Surg 2018;57(6):1200–3.
101. Valderrabano V, Hintermann B, Nigg BM, et al. Kinematic changes after fusion and total replacement of the ankle: part 1: Range of motion. Foot Ankle Int 2003;24(12):881–7.
102. DeSutter C, Dube V, Ross A, et al. Preliminary Experience With SPECT/CT to Evaluate Periarticular Arthritis Progression and the Relationship With Clinical Outcome Following Ankle Arthrodesis. Foot Ankle Int 2020;41(4):392–7.
103. Coester LM, Saltzman CL, Leupold J, et al. Long-term results following ankle arthrodesis for post-traumatic arthritis. J Bone Joint Surg Am 2001;83(2):219–28.
104. Klerken T, Kosse NM, Aarts CAM, et al. Long-term results after triple arthrodesis: Influence of alignment on ankle osteoarthritis and clinical outcome. Foot Ankle Surg 2019;25(2):247–50.
105. Rammelt S, Marti RK, Zwipp H. [Arthrodesis of the talonavicular joint]. Orthopade 2006;35(4):428–34.
106. Pagenstert GI, Hintermann B, Barg A, et al. Realignment surgery as alternative treatment of varus and valgus ankle osteoarthritis. Clin Orthop Relat Res 2007;462:156–68.
107. Thomas R, Daniels TR, Parker K. Gait analysis and functional outcomes following ankle arthrodesis for isolated ankle arthritis. J Bone Joint Surg Am 2006;88(3):526–35.
108. Zanolli DH, Nunley JA 2nd, Easley ME. Subtalar Fusion Rate in Patients With Previous Ipsilateral Ankle Arthrodesis. Foot Ankle Int 2015;36(9):1025–8.
109. Hintermann B, Barg A, Knupp M, et al. Conversion of painful ankle arthrodesis to total ankle arthroplasty. J Bone Joint Surg Am 2009;91(4):850–8.
110. Chu AK, Wilson MD, Houng B, et al. Outcomes of Ankle Arthrodesis Conversion to Total Ankle Arthroplasty: A Systematic Review. J Foot Ankle Surg 2021;60(2):362–7.
111. Davies MB, Rosenfeld PF, Stavrou P, et al. A comprehensive review of subtalar arthrodesis. Foot Ankle Int 2007;28(3):295–7.
112. Easley ME, Trnka HJ, Schon LC, et al. Isolated subtalar arthrodesis. J Bone Joint Surg Am 2000;82(5):613–24.
113. Ziegler P, Friederichs J, Hungerer S. Fusion of the subtalar joint for post-traumatic arthrosis: a study of functional outcomes and non-unions. Int Orthopaedics 2017;41(7):1387–93.
114. Lee W, Prat D, Wapner KL, et al. Comparison of 4 Different Fixation Strategies for Midfoot Arthrodesis: A Retrospective Comparative Study. Foot Ankle Spec 2021. 19386400211032482.
115. Füssenich W, Brusse-Keizer MGJ, Somford MP. Severe Hallux Valgus Angle Attended With High Incidence of Nonunion in Arthrodesis of the First Metatarsophalangeal Joint: A Follow-Up Study. J Foot Ankle Surg 2020;59(5):993–6.
116. Rammelt S, Panzner I, Mittlmeier T. Metatarsophalangeal Joint Fusion: Why and How? Foot Ankle Clin 2015;20(3):465–77.

First Metatarsophalangeal Arthrodesis for the Failed Hallux

Ahmed Khalil Attia, MD[a,*], Keith A. Heier, MD[b,1]

KEYWORDS

- Metatarsophalangeal joint arthrodesis • Revision metatarsophalangeal arthrodesis
- Hallux valgus • Hallux rigidus • Metatarsus primus elevatus
- Hallux avascular necrosis • Hallux infection

KEY POINTS

- Avoid plantar dissection of the first metatarsal to preserve vascularity. This is especially important in case of avascular necrosis caused by previous osteotomy.
- Plan ahead and anticipate first metatarsal shortening. Lesser metatarsal shortening osteotomy is commonly required to maintain the normal metatarsal cascade.
- Cup and cone reamers are excellent for joint preparation, but care should be practiced to avoid blowing up osteopenic metatarsal heads.
- Careful radiological and clinical evaluation of the sesamoid-metatarsal joint is strongly recommended, especially in cavus feet, hallux valgus, and revision surgeries. If sesamoidectomy is indicated, the flexor hallucis longus tendon should be preserved.
- Dorsal plates with a lag screw seem to provide superior biomechanical stability to crossed screws with similar union rates in hallux rigidus. However, in rheumatoid arthritis, hallux valgus, and osteopenic bone in general, dorsal locked plates are recommended.

INTRODUCTION

Hallux metatarsophalangeal joint (MTPJ) arthrodesis was first described in 1894 by Clutton, who recommended ankylosing the MTPJ to treat painful hallux valgus (HV). He used ivory pegs to stabilize the MTP joint. Surgeons over the last century have continuously modified the procedure and added indications other than HV to include hallux rigidus, rheumatoid arthritis, and revision of failed surgeries.

In this article, the authors address many common yet challenging clinical scenarios, and a few hot topics, related to hallux MTPJ arthrodesis. The authors aim to provide a

[a] Orthopedic Surgery and Rehabilitation Department, Penn State Milton S. Hershey Medical Center, Penn State College of Medicine, 500 University Drive, Hershey, PA 17033, USA;
[b] Orthotexas, Dallas, TX, USA
[1] Present address: 4780 North Josey Lane, Carrollton, TX 75010.
* Corresponding author.
E-mail address: Attia.footMD@gmail.com

Foot Ankle Clin N Am 27 (2022) 723–744
https://doi.org/10.1016/j.fcl.2022.07.001
1083-7515/22/© 2022 Elsevier Inc. All rights reserved.

foot.theclinics.com

condensed and evidence-based guide for some of the most challenging scenarios. They supplemented each section with a pearl box as a concise summary of the most salient points, an operative tip box, and radiographs of relevant cases.

METATARSALPHALANGEAL ARTHRODESIS IN METATARSUS PRIMUS ELEVATUS

The term metatarsus primus elevatus (MPE) has been first used in 1938 by Lambrinudi to describe the abnormally dorsally elevated first metatarsal head.[1] Since then, many authors discussed the role an elevated first metatarsal plays in the pathogenesis of hallux rigidus. Cheung and colleagues recently evaluated the foot alignment in 50 cases of symptomatic hallux rigidus compared with 50 controls using weight-bearing computed tomography scan (WBCT).[2] They reported that patients with hallux rigidus had MPE and that those with grade 3 and 4 had more MPE than those with grade 1 and 2 hallux rigidus.[2] Although there is a debate whether hallux rigidus is caused by MPE since the introduction of the term by Lambrinudi, MTPJ fusion with an elevated first metatarsal merits careful consideration of the fusion position.

Generally, the hallux MTPJ is preferably fused at a dorsiflexion angle to the position of the floor rather than the metatarsal, as the metatarsal declination varies, and the more predictable position would be with reference to the floor.[3] In the setting of a metatarsus primus elevatus, arthrodesis of the hallux MTP joint will result in a floating toe and ulceration of the toe tip from contact with shoes. Here, position of the fusion relative to the metatarsal may be in neutral alignment, but the hallux remains elevated relative to the floor. If MTPJ fusion is the only possible treatment option in the setting of a dorsiflexed first metatarsal, a plantarflexing osteotomy of the first metatarsal may be necessary before fusing the MTPJ (**Fig. 1**). Dorsiflexion at the MTPJ should be limited to a minimum or avoided all together. If the extensor hallucis longus tendon is tight, lengthening can be done to aid in bringing the toe down to the floor.[3]

MANAGEMENT OF SESAMOIDS IN METATARSALPHALANGEAL ARTHRODESIS

Sesamoids play an integral role in our understanding of the pathogenesis of hallux rigidus. The hallux MTPJ is considered a gliding hinge joint. The gliding of the metatarsal heads proximally on the sesamoids during gait allows for the axis of rotation to be shifted dorsally and proximally. When this gliding motion is blocked, the MTPJ is transformed into a simple hinge.[4] Moreover, the proximal displacement of the sesamoids represents the flexor hallucis longus (FHL) contracture in an attempt to stabilize the dysfunctional joint.[5] Although pain associated with hallux MTPJ arthritic changes can be effectively and reliably relieved with MTP fusion, this fusion simply does not address metatarso-sesamoid arthritis. Apart from arthritis, other etiologies of sesamoid-related plantar pain, such as stress fractures, sesamoiditis, osteomyelitis, and prominent hardware irritation, have also been reported.[6] The prevalence of arthritic changes of the metatarso-sesamoid joint remains under-reported. Doty and colleagues evaluated 39 cadaveric foot specimens for chondral damage of the MTPJ with HV. They reported that 74% of tibial sesamoids and 38% of fibular sesamoids had signs of articular erosions.[7]

Sesamoidectomy has been typically avoided due to the risk of subsequent deformity. However, this does not apply to hallux rigidus, where even total sesamoidectomy has been reported to have minimal morbidity even if the MTP joint was not fused. Tagoe and colleagues reported significant improvement in pain, function, footwear and MTP joint motion in 34 total sesamoidectomies for hallux rigidus at 2 years. They reported a median score of 90 on the AOFAS scale. None of their patients had

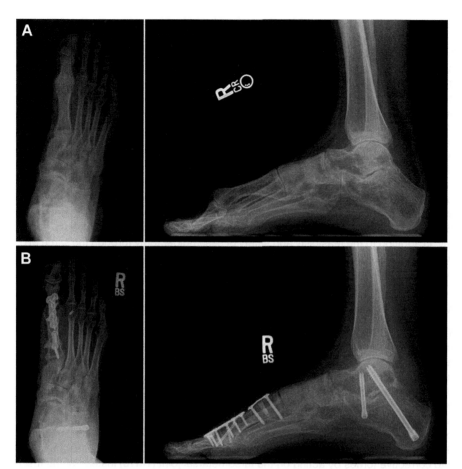

Fig. 1. Plain AP and lateral radiographs of pre (A) and postoperative (B) MTPJ and STJ arthrodesis. This 38-year-old man had advanced hallux rigidus and subtalar arthritis. An open wedge plantarflexing metatarsal osteotomy was done simultaneously to address the MPE.

subsequent transfer metatarsalgia, hallux malleolus, varus, or valgus.[8] The literature on the ideal management of the sesamoids in the context of hallux MTP fusion remains scarce and limited to case series with relatively small numbers of patients and no long-term follow-up. Tan and colleagues reported a case of persistent plantar pain caused by sesamoid-metatarsal arthritis 6 months after a successfully fused hallux MTPJ. Total sesamoidectomy, while preserving the FHL and FHB tendons, resulted in significant improvement.[9] Alshouli and colleagues reported a case series of simultaneous total sesamoidectomy and MTPJ arthrodesis with a dorsal plate.[10] Patients in their series were evaluated for metatarso-sesamoid arthritis using CT scan if they had pain with applied pressure against the sesamoid complex or degenerative changes of the sesamoid complex on AP or oblique radiographs. Five patients with grade III and IV hallux rigidus met these criteria for total sesamoidectomy. At 6 months postoperatively, all patients reported complete resolution of plantar pain. Similar to the 34 cases reported by Tagoe and colleagues,[8] no postoperative deformities or transfer metatarsalgia were reported.

Another recently reported option was incorporation of the metatarso-sesamoid joint in the MTPJ fusion surgery. Storts and colleagues reported on 97 MTPJ fusions where they routinely fused the sesamoids to the metatarsal heads.[11] They proposed that the added sesamoid joint preparation may have contributed to a high MTPJ fusion rate by increasing blood supply, but they did not test this hypothesis. Moreover, they did not evaluate the union of the sesamoid fusion, and no control group for sesamoid fusion was employed. While this is an interesting concept to discuss and a worthwhile research focus, surgeons should wait until this approach has undergone sufficient scientific scrutiny. The authors do not recommend this technique, because it may lead to a painful sesamoid fusion nonunion and one can still have the painful prominence of the sesamoids.

In conclusion, routine sesamoidectomy cannot be advised at the moment because of a lack of long-term outcomes studies and the modest level of evidence of available literature. However, in view of the high prevalence of metatarso-sesamoid degenerative changes, especially in advanced HV and cavus feet with a highly plantarflexed first ray, in addition to the feasibility and safety of sesamoidectomy through the same MTP fusion incision, the authors recommend sesamoidectomy as a part of MTPJ fusion when indicated in selected patients.

METATARSOPHALANGEAL JOINT ARTHRODESIS FOR HALLUX VALGUS

The ideal MTPJ-sparing management of severe HV remains a matter of debate. Double osteotomies,[12] proximal osteotomies,[13] and modified Lapidus procedure[14,15] have all been shown to be successful in the management of moderate-to-severe HV in the absence of MTPJ pathology, providing satisfactory MTPJ alignment while preserving the motion. However, indications for MTPJ arthrodesis include severe deformity, painful and limited MTPJ range of motion clinically and arthritis radiographically, rheumatoid arthritis, joint hypermobility, spasticity and progressive neurologic HV, and failed previous osteotomy surgery.[16–18] It was suggested that MTPJ fusion would transform the deforming forces from altered mechanics of flexor, adductor and extensor tendons into corrective forces by acting on the tarsometarsal joint (TMTJ) instead of the fused MTPJ[18] (Fig. 2).

Although many studies discussed the MTPJ arthrodesis in HV, most of them had their limitations. These limitations included varying age groups, reporting no functional outcomes,[18] and varying degrees of HV.[16,19–21] Moreover, some added a proximal metatarsal correction,[21] while others did not.[16,18–20] Nevertheless, all studies reported significant correction of the HV deformity using MTPJ arthrodesis. Coughlin and colleagues reported on 21 MTPJ fusions for idiopathic HV in patients 60 years and older with a mean follow-up of 8.2 years.[16] They performed MTPJ fusion for severe HV regardless of MTPJ degenerative changes, and for moderate HV with degenerative hallux MTPJ degeneration and lesser MTPJ instability. The mean preoperative 1- to 2-intermetatarsal angle (IMA) and HV angle (HVA) were 17.3° and 41.7°, respectively. The mean correction of IMA was 6.1°, while the HVA was corrected by 21.3°. Eighty percent of the patients reported excellent outcomes, while the remaining 20% reported good outcomes, with significant pain relief in 100% of the patients. McKean and colleagues reviewed 19 feet with only severe HV with a mean IMA of 19.2° and a mean HVA of 48.5°. They were able to achieve a mean correction of 8.3° and 36.4° to the IMA and HVA, respectively. In 37% of the feet with severe HV, the IMA was restored to normal (less than 9°). They proposed that an added proximal first metatarsal osteotomy is not required to achieve satisfactory HV deformity correction.[18]

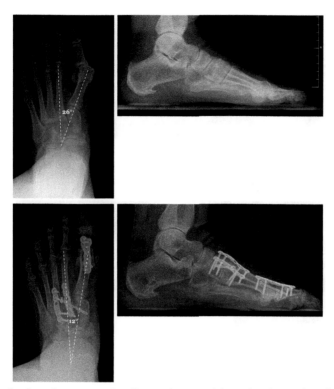

Fig. 2. Pre- (*top*) and postoperative (*bottom*) AP and lateral radiographs of 63-year-old woman with severe left HV (IMA = 26°, HVA = 40°) showing a 14° correction of the IMA after MTPJ arthrodesis (dorsal plate + compression screw). Calcaneal bone graft was used for the 2-3TMT fusion. A first TMT fusion was avoided to help maintain a more flexible first ray.

On the other hand, Rippstein and colleagues added a proximal correction in the form of either a Mau osteotomy or a modified Lapidus procedure in their series of 18 MTPJ arthrodeses for severe HV.[21] The proximal correction was added if the IMA was more than 10° after MTPJ fusion. The combined procedure achieved a mean correction of 14 and 40.2 in IMA and HVA, respectively. In all the patients, a normal IMA angle (<9°) was achieved. There was no statistically significant difference in correction between Mau osteotomy and modified Lapidus groups. Although no nonunion, malunion, significant first ray shortening, or transfer metatarsalgia were reported in their series, these complications are known to potentially arise from proximal correction osteotomies and should be used judiciously when indicated.[22] This is an excellent strategy to correct the deformity, but it certainly adds the potential for more surgical complications and necessitates limited weightbearing. The ability to have full weightbearing in a boot was one of the benefits of doing the fusion for an elderly patient with a severe bunion (**Fig. 3**).

A recent alternative to proximal bony correction is the use of a miniature suture button system.[23–25] Gonzales and colleagues reported on combined distal soft tissue procedures combined with proximal suture button suspension in 22 feet with HV.[23] They achieved a mean reduction of the IMA and HVA of 11.7° and 22.8°, respectively. Having this technique in the toolbox can prove useful as an adjunct to MTP fusion to further improve the IMA correction without further shortening the first ray by added proximal bony correction. Moreover, this metatarsal suspension technique requires

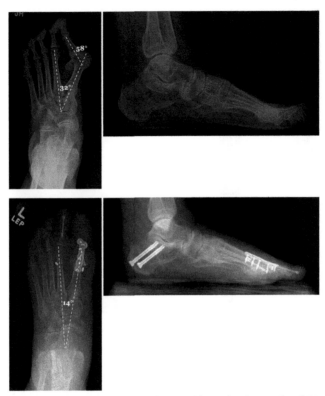

Fig. 3. Pre- (*top*) and postoperative (*bottom*) AP and lateral radiographs of 71-year-old man with severe right HV (IMA = 11°, HVA = 75°) showing a 58° correction of the HVA and 5° correction of the IMA using MTPJ arthrodesis (dorsal plate + compression screw) and suture button suspension. Weil osteotomies were also performed to help reduce the MTP joints.

smaller incisions, allows earlier weight bearing, and shortens the recovery time.[23] However, this relatively new technique comes with its own set of complications such as second metatarsal fractures, either intraoperatively or later as stress fractures.[23] Additionally, there are no long-term outcome studies reported to date, and the evidence is limited to small series.[23–25] (**Fig. 4**).

Finally, it is crucial to understand that MTPJ fusion is not an alternative to proper soft tissue balancing done with MTPJ-sparing procedures to avoid recurrence and malunion. Moreover, nonunion of MTPJ fusion is significantly higher in HV than in hallux rigidus, 14% and 0%, respectively.[26] Hence respecting the soft tissues, using appropriately solid implants, and avoiding heat necrosis while preparing the MTPJ should always be kept in mind. When MTPJ fusion is not sufficient to correct the IMA, a TMTJ arthrodesis can be added.[3]

METATARSOPHALANGEAL JOINT ARTHRODESIS IN HALLUX VALGUS INTERPHALANGEUS

HV interphalangeus (HVI) can be corrected during MTPJ arthrodesis by making the proximal phalanx cut parallel to the IPJ and using an oblique medial cut of the metatarsal head. This might lead to significant shortening of the hallux; length can be restored by adding a bone block to the MTPJ arthrodesis (**Fig. 5**).

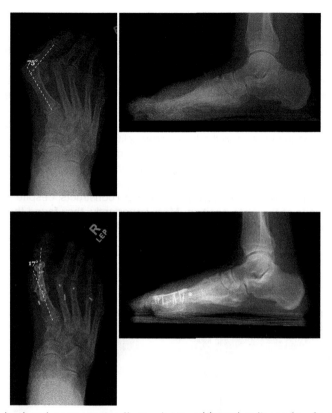

Fig. 4. Pre- (*top*) and postoperative (*bottom*) AP and lateral radiographs of a 64 year old woman with severe left HV (IMA = 32°, HVA = 58°) showing an 18° correction of the IMA with a combined MTPJ arthrodesis (dorsal plate + compression screw) and suture button suspension.

If symptomatic HVI occurs after MTPJ arthrodesis, remove the plate/screw construct and perform a medially based closing wedge osteotomy to correct the deformity if the MTPJ fusion has already united. If the MTPJ fusion is not completely healed, the surgeon could replace a plate or a lag screw back across the MTPJ for extra stability and protection.

IMPLANT CONSIDERATIONS FOR METATARSOPHALANGEAL JOINT ARTHRODESIS

The ideal implant for MTP arthrodesis, and for many foot and ankle procedures, has been a matter of debate. Implants for MTP fusion evolved from ivory pegs in the 1890s to include Kirschner wires, Steinman pins, memory staples, screws, and plates.[27] This debate is expected to persist as newer implants enter the market, generating discussion and further research. For the sake of simplicity, implants can be broadly classified into compression screws or plates. Plates in turn can be straight or precontoured with variable dorsiflexion angles, locked or static, and have variable geometries and materials. A combination of a dorsal plate and a compression screw across the fusion has also been recently described.[28] The authors will discuss the available literature on different implants across 3 main domains: biomechanics, clinical outcomes, and cost.

Biomechanics

One notable difference of MTP plating compared with most orthopedic applications is that plates in the former are applied to the compression side rather than the conventional tension side in the latter.[29] An ideal position would be a plantar position that is limited by the anatomy of the hallux, placing the dorsal plate in a mechanical disadvantageous position.[30] More importantly, the quality of the bone (ie, bone mineral density) also plays a crucial role in stability.

The bone in HV is generally osteopenic compared with the sclerotic nature of hallux rigidus. Matching the implant to the bone personality is crucial.[31]

Neufeld and colleagues compared a cannulated crossed screw construct versus a dorsal neutralization plate with a 0.062 oblique Kirschner wire construct in 14 matched cadaveric specimens.[30] They concluded that the plantar load to 1 mm displacement and failure (2 mm displacement) were similar for both constructs, despite the mechanical disadvantage of the plate position. More importantly, they found that the screw construct failed through fracturing the bone while the predominant mode of failure of the plate construct was bending of the plate (79%). Even after the plate was bent, some rigidity remained.

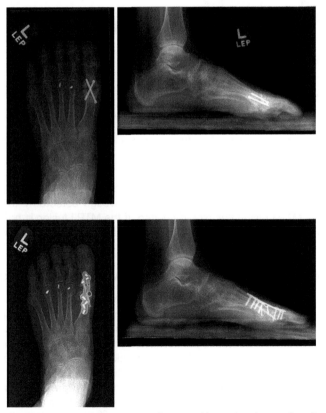

Fig. 7. Pre- (top) and postoperative (bottom) AP and lateral radiographs of a failed MTP fusion with crossing lag screws in a 65-year-old man. Allograft bone block and dorsal plate used for revision fusion because of bone loss at the joint nonunion site.

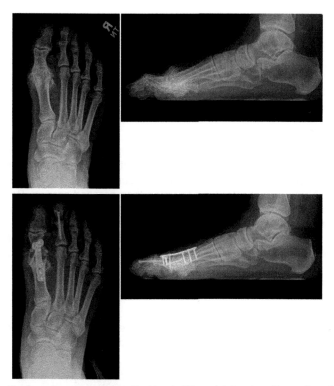

Fig. 5. Pre- (*top*) and postoperative (*bottom*) AP and lateral radiographs of first MTPJ arthrodesis with bone block allograft. This 60-year-old man had severe hallux rigidus with HVI.

Cone and colleagues showed that adding a lag screw to the dorsal titanium locked compression plate construct significantly increases the rigidity of the construct while not increasing the union rates in a total of 99 consecutive MTP fusions.[28] The dorsiflexion angle at final follow-up (12 months) increased by a mean of 0.6° in the plate and lag screw group in comparison to 6.7° with the plate alone, showing that adding a lag screw helps maintain the immediate postoperative sagittal alignment. Hunt and colleagues found that a titanium locked plate led to higher union in rheumatoid arthritis patients than a nonlocked stainless steel plate.[32]

A notable biomechanical study by Fuld and colleagues compared 2 crossed fully threaded screws to a dorsal locked plate with a compression screw construct in 18 matched cadaveric specimen pairs that they loaded 250,000 cycles to simulate walking in a short leg cast for 6 weeks.[31] They concluded that despite the significantly higher stiffness of the screws construct, the ultimate load to failure was almost equal. They also measured the bone mineral density of the specimens and found a strong correlation with load to failure in the screw group but no correlation in the plate group. Again, highlighting that a plate and a screw construct would be a superior option for osteopenic bone. Other patient factors were predictors of failure with screws but not with plates, such as metatarsal midshaft width on anteroposterior (AP) and lateral radiographs. They also recommended the use of fully threaded screws if a crossed screw construct is used.[31] In a similar study, Harris and colleagues found partially threaded crossed screws to be about 50% less stiff in comparison to plates, with an equivalent maximum load to failure.[33] Other studies found a dorsal plate with a lag screw to be stiffer with a higher load to failure than crossed screws for MTP fusion.[34–36]

To sum up, it appears that the dorsal plate with a lag screw is biomechanically equivalent, if not superior, to the crossed screw construct. Fully threaded screws are superior to partially threaded ones,[37] and locking plates are superior to nonlocking plates.[38]

Clinical Outcomes

Excellent outcomes of modern dorsal plates with supplementary lag screw fixation of the MTP fusion have been reported. However, most studies have shown that the potential biomechanical superiority of the plate and screw construct did not translate to a higher union rate or a shorter time to union than crossed screws. Both implants resulted in comparable and excellent clinical outcomes.[28,39–41] Unfortunately, there is a marked heterogeneity in the literature in implant design, indications, patient demographics and comorbidities, operative technique, postoperative protocols, surgeon experience, and small numbers of patients. Consequently, solid conclusions about the superiority of an implant are not realistic. Large standardized multicentric studies are required.

Cost

Hyer and colleagues[27] retrospectively compared the crude cost of crossed compression screws (n = 14) versus 5-hole titanium dorsal low profile precontoured

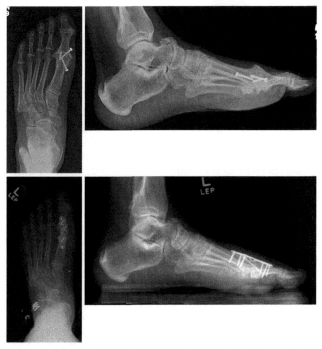

Fig. 6. Pre- (*top*) and postoperative (*bottom*) AP and lateral radiographs of a 59-year-old man with failed MTP fusion with crossing lag screws. Revision fusion with an allograft bone block and a dorsal plate because of poor bone quality at the joint level and loss of bone with removal of the screws.

compression plates (n = 37) in outpatient primary MTPJ arthrodesis. They concluded that the mean implant cost of the screws contrast was $374.05 plus or minus $76.30 while the dorsal plate construct mean implant cost was $603.57 plus or minus $234.70, with a strong statistically significant difference. They added that there were no statistically significant differences in union rate, time to union, and complication rates between both groups. Although this study can help with cost analysis of the implant only, the study had some limitations to its clinical application. First the study was underpowered to detect differences in nonunion (1 case in either group). They also analyzed only the implant cost rather than a comprehensive cost analysis. They only included primary MTP fusion and excluded neuropathic, diabetic, revision, infection, and active smokers, which further limits its clinical application.

In summary, despite their higher cost, modern dorsal locked plates with a compression screw across the fusion site are increasingly recognized as a reliable implant for MTP arthrodesis, especially in osteopenic bone and older patients. They also allow using a bone block to restore the length of the hallux. However, there is no level I evidence to support their superiority over 2 crossed fully threaded compression

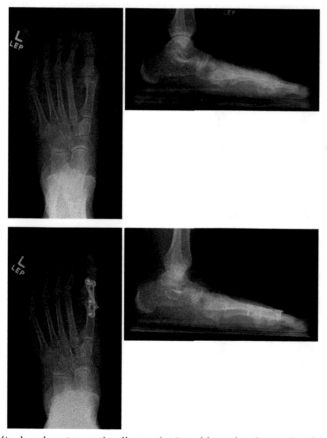

Fig. 8. Pre- (*top*) and postoperative (*bottom*) AP and lateral radiographs of a 62-year-old man with a failed Cartiva implant with subsidence of the implant and persistent pain. Contrary to previous studies, a bone block allograft with dorsal plate had to be used for the revision fusion because of significant bone loss and shortening at the joint.

screws that provide similar fusion rates at a lower cost. The implant choice should be tailored to patient needs, indication, bone quality, availability, and surgeon's experience. The authors routinely use the locked plate/screw construct with a lag screw as they find this leads to more predictable alignment and outcomes (**Figs. 6** and **7**).

MANAGEMENT OF COMPLICATIONS OF METATARSOPHALANGEAL JOINT ARTHRODESIS
In Situ Versus Bone Block Graft for Revision Metatarsophalangeal Joint Arthrodesis

Although mild shortening of the hallux with in situ MTP fusion is well tolerated functionally and cosmetically, many indications for MTP arthrodesis are associated with significant bone loss that render in situ fusion prone to significant shortening of the hallux leading to a floating toe and transfer metatarsalgia. Bone block augmented MTP fusion to lengthen the hallux is indicated if the bone loss exceeds 0.5 to 1 cm.[3,42] Failed resection and hemi and total MTP arthroplasties often result in bone loss that is significant enough to require hallux lengthening with bone blocks (**Figs. 8** and **9**).

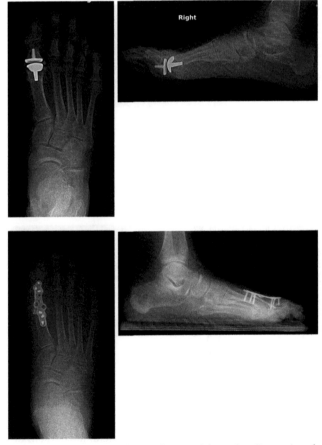

Fig. 9. Pre- (*top*) and postoperative (*bottom*) AP and lateral radiographs of a 72-year-old woman with a stiff and painful and loose total toe replacement. MTP fusion revision with dorsal plate and an allograft bone block spacer.

Another potential cause for challenging bone defects is avascular necrosis (AVN), which is discussed later. However, the management of bone defects caused by AVN follows the same principles.[42,43]

Many options for bone grafts are available. Autografts are biologically superior, readily available, and do not involve added costs but require an added surgical procedure with potential morbidity.[42] Iliac crest auto and allografts and femoral allografts have been used. Commercial synthetic grafts are also available. Distal lower extremity autografts such as calcaneal, proximal, and distal tibial autografts have also been successfully used for foot and ankle procedures. The postoperative immobilization and non-weight bearing will typically include the distal lower extremity graft donor site, possibly avoiding added interference with activities of daily living other than those of the fusion surgery. The grafts may also be readily available within the surgical field, with an overall complication rate as low as 2.43% compared with 19.3% in iliac crest autografts.[44–46] However, the graft preparation is more important than the graft source to allow the ideal final alignment of the hallux.

In the authors' experience, allografts may work equal or better in older patients with poor bone quality. The precut, presized allograft pieces work well for this problem. The authors typically soak the bulk allograft in the patient's blood or iliac crest bone marrow aspirate concentrate (BMAC) and can supplement the fusion, especially in

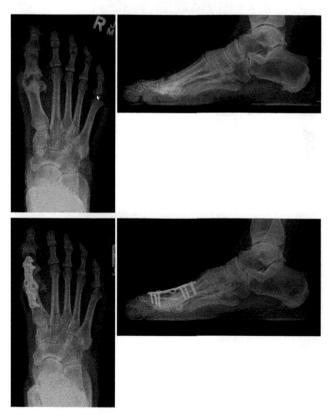

Fig. 10. Plain AP and lateral radiographs of pre- (*top*) and post- (*bottom*) MTPJ arthrodesis with interposition bone block. This 54-year-old woman had AVN after a cheilectomy and drilling of a metatarsal osteochondral defect (OCD) 2 years before the fusion.

the cases of greater than 10 mm of defect, with calcaneal or tibial cancellous bone or demineralized bone matrix (DBM).

Managing Avascular Necrosis: In Situ Fusion Versus Bone Block Graft

AVN of the first metatarsal head has been reported to complicate distal and diaphyseal osteotomies of the hallux metatarsal due to disruption of the intraosseous blood supply.[47,48] The only remaining blood supply to the metatarsal head is the plexus formed by the first dorsal metatarsal, first plantar metatarsal, and medial plantar arteries at the plantar lateral neck of the metatarsal. Hence, avoiding aggressive plantar dissection of the plantar neck at the level of capsular insertion is crucial to avoid AVN as recommended by Molloy and Widnall.[49] However, AVN of the first metatarsal head has also been reported to occur spontaneously.[50,51]

AVN can be asymptomatic with subtle radiographic changes, but it can also be severe with significant collapse of the subchondral bone, fragmentation of the metatarsal head, and MTPJ degeneration with severe pain and limitation. Furthermore, the hallux is shortened, and transfer metatarsalgia will occur. At this stage, the only management option is MTPJ arthrodesis. However, the size of the avascular

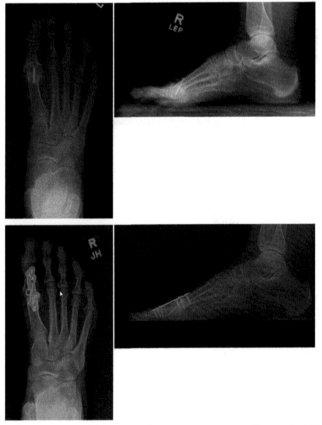

Fig. 11. Plain AP and lateral radiographs of pre- (*top*) and post- (*bottom*) MTPJ arthrodesis with interposition bone block. This 56-year-old woman had AVN after distal metatarsal osteotomy for mild hallux rigidus and HV.

bone to be removed could further shorten the hallux.[47] Using bone block grafts is required in most cases to restore the length of the first ray, as discussed earlier (**Figs. 10** and **11**).

Although bone block lengthening seems the logical choice, the underlying cause for the AVN is a crucial variable to consider. AVN precipitated by hallux lengthening that compromised the vascularity adds complexity to the management. Debridement of the avascular bone can leave a large defect that would otherwise require a bone block distraction arthrodesis, leading to lengthening of the hallux that precipitated the AVN in the first place. Hence, it is reasonable to accept limited lengthening of the hallux length or even shorten it further and opting for shortening of the lesser metatarsals to restore the cascade.[52] Avoid using a tourniquet in MTPJ fusion procedures for

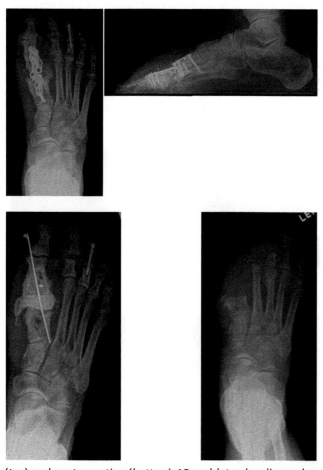

Fig. 12. Pre- (*top*) and postoperative (*bottom*) AP and lateral radiographs of a 61-year-old man. He had a chevron osteotomy that developed severe AVN. He subsequently had 2 attempts at an MTP fusion, one with an allograft and one with an autograft bulk ICBG. None of the fusions healed, and he was eventually noted to have a chronic infection and unhealthy bone. He was treated with a cement antibiotic spacer to help eradicate the infection, but he eventually chose to have a first ray amputation (bottom right).

AVN to better judge the vascularity. Judiciously and safely lengthen the hallux to preserve the vascularity and avoid nonunion and AVN.

Managing Infection with Cement Spacer

Managing periprosthetic infection using staged revisions with cement spacers has been the standard of care in total hip and knee replacements. However, there is little reported on the use of cement spacers in infected MTPJ prosthetic replacement and arthrodesis. Uncontrolled diabetes and vascular insufficiency can make preventing and managing infections a daunting task, and amputation is not uncommon despite best efforts (**Fig. 12**). Hallux amputations start a vicious circle of transfer metatarsalgia, ulcerations, infections, and further forefoot reamputations.[53] Therefore, every attempt should be made to eradicate the infection while preserving the hallux. Antibiotic impregnated cement spacers allow local delivery of high concentrations of antibiotics for 8 or more weeks.[54] Spacers also provide stability to promote healing, as defects created by debridement of infected bone can result in instability.[55] These spacers can be used a bridge to a second procedure after resolution of the infection or left permanently in place.[56]

Myerson and colleagues reported on 5 cases of MTPJ infection following hallux valgus surgeries treated with staged revision with tobramycin-impregnated bone cement.[55] Four of these cases had osteomyelitis in addition to MTPJ septic arthritis. The spacer was left in place for 3 to 6 weeks, and patients received intravenous

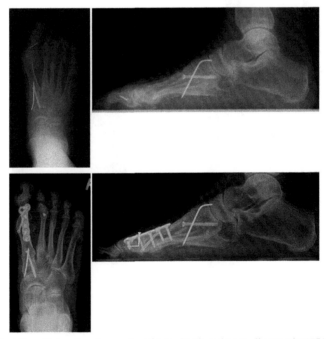

Fig. 13. Plain AP and lateral radiographs of pre- (*top*) and post- (*bottom*) MTPJ arthrodesis. This 63-year-old woman had hallux rigidus and residual HV after a previous Akin osteotomy and Lapidus. An MTP joint fusion was performed for a refractory bunion with arthritis rather than doing a revision Lapidus. The patient chose the MTP fusion, because it allowed immediate weightbearing and significantly eliminated the potential of a persistently painful MTP joint with the potential of a recurrent bunion.

antibiotics. The second stage involved removal of the spacer and iliac crest bone block MTPJ arthrodesis. Infection resolved in all the cases, and no amputations were required. Four patients went onto fusion, and 1 patient had asymptomatic pseudoarthrosis.[55] Melamed and Peled described a series of 23 cases of diabetic forefoot infections treated with gentamicin with or without vancomycin-impregnated polymethylmethacrylate spacers. Twenty-one (91.3%) infections resolved, and only 2 patients (6.7%) required amputations to control the infection.[56]

HALLUX METATARSOPHALANGEAL ARTHRODESIS WITH AN ALREADY FUSED TARSOMETATARSAL JOINT

First TMTJ arthrodesis is a common and successful procedure for HV deformity correction, especially with an unstable medial column. Hallux rigidus following a TMTJ fusion is can be challenging. MTPJ arthrodesis with an already fused TMTJ creates a stiff medial column, with significant forces placed on the proximal interphalangeal joint (PIPJ). Another variable to be considered is the flexion angle at which the TMTJ is fused. If the TMTJ is fused in excessive plantarflexion, a dorsal closing wedge osteotomy might be needed to avoid forefoot supination, keratosis under the metatarsal head, and limitation of the toe-off. Conversely, if the TMTJ is fused in excessive dorsiflexion, a plantarflexing opening wedge osteotomy might be needed to avoid

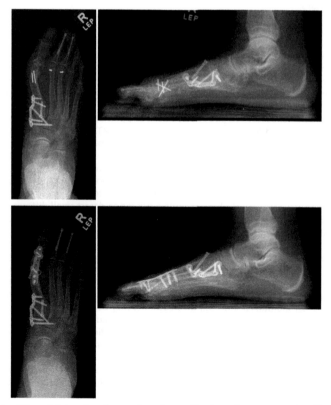

Fig. 14. Plain AP and lateral radiographs of pre- (*top*) and postoperative (*bottom*) MTPJ arthrodesis. This 58-year-old woman had severe hallux rigidus after a previous metatarsal osteotomy and TMTJ fusion for HV.

floating toe and transfer metatarsalgia (**Figs. 13** and **14**). Tibial sesamoidectomy can also be added to reduce the risk of plantar pain caused by the now stiffer medial column. Also, the MTPJ should be fused in slight dorsiflexion rather than flat. Consider excising the tibial sesamoid as the first ray will be stiff, and patients will be more likely to have pain under the MTP joint, as discussed previously.

HALLUX METATARSOPHALANGEAL JOINT ARTHRODESIS WITH AN ALREADY FUSED INTERPHALANGEAL JOINT

Degenerative changes of the MTPJ in the presence of an already fused IPJ is extremely challenging to manage with fusion. This is often not well tolerated since patients will likely complain that the toe sticks up too much with increased pressure under the MTPJ if the IPJ is fused in dorsiflexion. If the IPJ was fused in some degree of plantarflexion, a painful callous at the tip of the toe or over the dorsal IP joint may be present. MTPJ motion-preserving procedures such as interposition arthroplasty, prosthetic replacement, resection arthroplasty, or resurfacing should be strongly considered instead of MTPJ fusion.

CLINICS CARE POINTS

Pearls and Pitfalls
- Avoid MTP dorsiflexion in metatarsus primus elevatus to avoid a floating toe and pain under the sesamoids. A plantarflexing metatarsal osteotomy plus or minus extensor hallucis longus (EHL) tendon lengthening can help bring the toe to the floor.
- Clinically and radiologically evaluate the metatarso-sesamoid complex preoperatively and carefully inspect the sesamoids at the time of the MTP fusion surgery. When arthritic changes are present, sesamoidectomy should be considered in the index fusion surgery rather than subjecting the patient to another surgery should planter pain remain after fusion.
- MTPJ arthrodesis for severe HV (IMA >16°, HVA >40°) provides a solid deformity correction and good to excellent functional outcomes, especially in MTPJ arthritic changes, rheumatoid arthritis, and revision surgery. Additional proximal correction can be utilized for additional IMA correction. However, finding a balance between IMA correction and avoiding complications of the additional proximal procedure is recommended.
- A hybrid dorsal locked plate and a lag screw construct are biomechanically equivalent, if not superior, to crossed lag screws for MTP arthrodesis. Union rates and time to union are similar in both constructs; however, studies are underpowered to detect small differences. The authors recommend the hybrid plate construct in HV, older patients, osteopenic bone, and revision cases.
- When the expected hallux shortening exceeds 1 cm, adding a bone block to the fusion to restore the length and avoid transfer metatarsalgia is required. If adequate lengthening is limited by the hallux vascularity, shortening osteotomies of the lesser toes are advised.
- Severe AVN with metatarsal head collapse usually requires excision of a large area of necrotic bone, necessitating bone block MTPJ arthrodesis. When lengthening is limited by the vascularity, lesser metatarsal shortening osteotomies may be indicated.
- In cases of infection, every attempt to preserve the hallux should be made. Antibiotic impregnated cement spacers can be a valuable tool to eradicate the infection while providing stability to promote healing. However, amputations will inevitably be required in some cases.
- Consider the position of the TMTJ fusion when planning the MTPJ fusion. Dorsi or plantarflexing osteotomies can be added to allow for proper first ray alignment. When both the TMTJ and MTPJ fusions are done right, the procedure can be well tolerated despite the stiff medial column.
- MTPJ arthrodesis with an already fused IPJ is poorly tolerated. MTPJ motion-preserving procedures should be considered instead of arthrodesis

Operative Tips

- MPE: If the first metatarsal is mildly elevated, and there is some flexibility at the first TMT joint, the alignment could be managed at the first MTP joint with the fusion. If the first metatarsal is significantly elevated, then do the osteotomy before the toe fusion. The osteotomy could be done at the same time as the MTP fusion, or before the fusion if there are bone and soft tissue healing concerns.
- Sesamoids: The tibial sesamoid is often symptomatic and could be removed at the time of the index procedure through the same dorsal incision. Elevate the metatarsal head with a bone hook or clamp, and then shell out the sesamoid(s) with careful attention to leaving the FHL tendon intact.
- Short hallux revision: After preparing the fusion site down to bleeding bone, use a laminar spreader to distract the fusion site until desired hallux length is achieved. If using a tourniquet, deflate it to confirm that the toe vascularity is not compromised by the distraction. Reduce the distraction gradually, if necessary, until the vascularity is satisfactory, then measure the gap. The bone block is then fashioned to fit this gap. If the hallux is still short, lesser metatarsal osteotomy can restore the metatarsal cascade and minimize transfer metatarsalgia.
- Infection: Err on the side of more bone resection, getting back to healthy bleeding bone is necessary for a successful fusion. Plan ahead for a potential bone block fusion to accommodate increased and unexpected bone resection

DISCLOSURE

A.K. Attia: Nothing to disclose. K.A. Heier: Royalties from I2Bone. Stock ownership 4Web, I2B.

REFERENCES

1. Lambrinudi C. Metatarsus primus elevatus. Proc R Soc Med 1938;31:1273.
2. Cheung ZB, Myerson MS, Tracey J, et al. Weightbearing CT scan assessment of foot alignment in patients with hallux rigidus. Foot Ankle Int 2018;39(1):67–74.
3. Myerson MS, Kadakia AR. 27 - Arthrodesis of the hallux metatarsophalangeal and interphalangeal joints. In: Myerson MS, Kadakia AR, editors. Reconstructive foot and ankle surgery: management of complications. 3rd edition. Elsevier; 2019. p. 411–38. https://doi.org/10.1016/B978-0-323-49693-3.00027-5.
4. Roukis TS, Scherer PR, Anderson CF. Position of the first ray and motion of the first metatarsophalangeal joint. JAPMA 1996;86(11):538–46.
5. Shamus J, Shamus E, Gugel RN, et al. The effect of sesamoid mobilisation, flexor hallucis strengthening, and gait training on reducing pain and restoring function in individuals with hallux limitus: a clinical trial. J Orthop Sports Phys Ther 2004; 34:7368–76.
6. Richardson EG. Hallucal sesamoid pain: causes and surgical treatment. J Am Acad Orthop Surg 1999;7:270–8.
7. Doty JF, Coughlin MJ, Schutt S, et al. Articular chondral damage of the first metatarsal head and sesamoids: analysis of cadaver hallux valgus. Foot Ankle Int 2013;34(8):1090–6.
8. Tagoe M, Brown HA, Rees SM. Total sesamoidectomy for painful hallux rigidus: a medium-term outcome study. Foot Ankle Int 2009;30:640–6.
9. Tan J, Lau JTC. Metatarso-sesamoid osteoarthritis as a cause of pain after first metatarsophalangeal joint fusion: Case report. Foot Ankle Int 2011;32(8):822–5.
10. Alshouli MT, Lin A, Kadakia AR. Simultaneous first metatarsophalangeal joint arthrodesis and sesamoidectomy with a single dorsomedial incision. Foot Ankle Spec 2014;7(5):403–8.

11. Storts EC, Camasta CA. Immediate weightbearing of first metatarsophalangeal joint fusion comparing buried crossed kirschner wires versus crossing screws: does incorporating the sesamoids into the fusion contribute to higher incidence of bony union? J Foot Ankle Surg 2016;55(3):562–6.

12. Braito M, Dammerer D, Hofer-Picout P, et al. Proximal opening wedge osteotomy with distal chevron osteotomy of the first metatarsal for the treatment of moderate to severe hallux valgus. Foot Ankle Int 2019;40:89–97.

13. Faber FW, van Kampen PM, Bloembergen MW. Long-term results of the Hohmann and Lapidus procedure for the correction of hallux valgus: a prospective, randomized trial with eight- to 11-year follow-up involving 101 feet. Bone Joint J 2013;95-B:1222–6.

14. Ellington JK, Myerson MS, Coetzee JC, et al. The use of the Lapidus procedure for recurrent hallux valgus. Foot Ankle Int 2011;32:674–80.

15. Coetzee JC, Resig SG, Kuskowski M, et al. The Lapidus procedure as salvage after failed surgical treatment of hallux valgus: a prospective cohort study. J Bone Joint Surg Am 2003;85:60–5.

16. Coughlin MJ, Grebing BR, Jones CP. Arthrodesis of the first metatarsophalangeal joint for idiopathic hallux valgus: inter- mediate results. Foot Ankle Int 2005;26(10):783–92.

17. Shi GG, Whalen JL, Turner NS, et al. Operative approach to adult hallux valgus deformity: principles and techniques. J Am Acad Orthop Surg 2020;28(10):410–8.

18. McKean RM, Bergin PF, Watson G, et al. Radiographic evaluation of intermetatarsal angle correction following first MTP joint arthrodesis for severe hallux valgus. Foot Ankle Int 2016;37(11):1183–6.

19. Cronin JJ, Limbers JP, Kutty S, et al. Intermetatarsal angle after first metatarsophalangeal joint arthrodesis for hallux valgus. Foot Ankle Int 2006;27(2):104–9.

20. Pydah SK, Toh EM, Sirikonda SP, et al. Intermetatarsal angular change following fusion of the first metatarsophalangeal joint. Foot Ankle Int 2009;30(5):415–8.

21. Rippstein PF, Park YU, Naal FD. Combination of first metatarsophalangeal joint arthrodesis and proximal correction for severe hallux valgus deformity. Foot Ankle Int 2012;33(5):400–5.

22. Mann RA, Rudicel S, Graves SC. Repair of hallux valgus with a distal soft-tissue procedure and proximal metatarsal osteotomy. A long-term follow-up. Bone Joint Surg 1992;74(1):124–9.

23. Gonzalez TA, Smith JT, Bluman EM, et al. Treatment of hallux valgus deformity using a suture button device: a preliminary report. Foot Ankle Orthop 2018;3(4). 247301141880695.

24. Holmes GB, Hsu AR. Correction of intermetatarsal angle in hallux valgus using small suture button device. Foot Ankle Int 2013;34(4):543–9.

25. Ponnapula P, Wittock R. Application of an interosseous suture and button device for hallux valgus correction: a review of outcomes in a small series. J Foot Ankle Surg 2010;49(2):159.e21-6.

26. Korim MT, Allen PE. Effect of pathology on union of first metatarsophalangeal joint arthrodesis. Foot Ankle Int 2015;36(1):51–4.

27. Hyer CF, Glover JP, Berlet GC, et al. Cost comparison of crossed screws versus dorsal plate construct for first metatarsophalangeal joint arthrodesis. J Foot Ankle Surg 2008;47(1):13–8.

28. Cone B, Staggers JR, Naranje S, et al. First metatarsophalangeal joint arthrodesis: does the addition of a lag screw to a dorsal locking plate influence union rate and/or final alignment after fusion. J Foot Ankle Surg 2018;57(2):259–63.

29. Muller ME, Allgower M, Schneider R, et al. Manual of Internal fixation. Berlin: Springer-Verlag; 1970.
30. Neufeld SK, Parks BG, Naseef GS, et al. Arthrodesis of the first metatarsophalangeal joint: A biomechanical study comparing memory compression staples, cannulated screws, and a dorsal plate. Foot Ankle Int 2002;23(2):97–101.
31. Fuld RS, Kumparatana P, Kelley J, et al. Biomechanical comparison of low-profile contoured locking plate with single compression screw to fully threaded compression screws for first MTP fusion. Foot Ankle Int 2019;40(7):836–44.
32. Hunt KJ, Ellington JK, Anderson RB, et al. Locked versus nonlocked plate fixation for hallux MTP arthrodesis. Foot Ankle Int 2011;32(7):704–9.
33. Harris E, Moroney P, Tourne Y. Arthrodesis of the first metatarsophalangeal joint—a biomechanical comparison of four fixation techniques. Foot Ankle Surg 2017; 23(4):268–74.
34. Buranosky DJ, Taylor DT, Sage RA, et al. First metatarsophalangeal joint arthrodesis: quantitative mechanical testing of six-hole dorsal plate versus crossed screw fixation in cadaveric specimens. J Foot Ankle Surg 2001;40(4):208–13.
35. Campbell B, Schimoler P, Belagaje S, et al. Weight-bearing recommendations after first metatarsophalangeal joint arthrodesis fixation: a biomechanical comparison. J Orthop Surg Res 2017;12(1):23.
36. Politi J, Hayes J, Njus G, et al. First metatarsal-phalangeal joint arthrodesis: a biomechanical assessment of stability. Foot Ankle Int 2003;24:332–7.
37. Lucas KJ, Morris RP, Buford WL Jr, et al. Biomechanical comparison of first metatarsophalangeal joint arthrodeses using triple-threaded headless screws versus partially threaded lag screws. Foot Ankle Surg 2014;20(2):144–8.
38. Hunt KJ, Barr CR, Lindsey DP, et al. Locked versus nonlocked plate fixation for first metatarsophalangeal arthrodesis: a biomechanical investigation. Foot Ankle Int 2012;33(11):984–90.
39. Kumar S, Pradhan R, Rosenfeld PF. First metatarsophalangeal arthrodesis using a dorsal plate and a compression screw. Foot Ankle Int 2010;31(9):797–801.
40. Hyer CF, Scott RT, Swiatek M. A Retrospective comparison of four plate constructs for first metatarsophalangeal joint fusion: static plate, static plate with lag screw, locked plate, and locked plate with lag screw. J Foot Ankle Surg 2012;51(3):285–7.
41. Dening J, van Erve RHGP. Arthrodesis of the first metatarsophalangeal joint: a retrospective analysis of plate versus screw fixation. J Foot Ankle Surg 2012; 51(2):172–5.
42. Schuh R, Trnka HJ. First metatarsophalangeal arthrodesis for severe bone loss. Foot Ankle Clin 2011;16(1):13–20.
43. Whalen J. Clinical tip: interpositional bone graft for first MP fusion. Foot Ankle Int 2009;30(2):160–2.
44. Attia AK, Mahmoud K, ElSweify K, et al. Donor site morbidity of calcaneal, distal tibial, and proximal tibial cancellous bone autografts in foot and ankle surgery. A systematic review and meta-analysis of 2296 bone grafts. Foot Ankle Surg 2021;(21):S1268–7731, 00201-0.
45. Cross DJ, DiDomenico LA. Calcaneal bone graft procedures: an analysis of post-surgical complications. J Foot Ankle Surg 2019;58(4):730–3.
46. Dimitriou R, Mataliotakis GI, Angoules AG, et al. Complications following autologous bone graft harvesting from the iliac crest and using the RIA: a systematic review. Injury 2011;42(suppl 2):S3–15.

47. Filippi J, Briceno J. Complications after metatarsal osteotomies for hallux valgus: malunion, nonunion, avascular necrosis, and metatarsophalangeal osteoarthritis. Foot Ankle Clin 2020;25(1):169–82.
48. Gurevich M, Bialik V, Eidelman M, et al. Avascular necrosis of the 1st metatarsal head. Acta Chir Orthop Traumatol Cech 2008;75(5):396–8.
49. Molloy A, Widnall J. Scarf osteotomy. Foot Ankle Clin 2014;19:165–80.
50. Fu FH, Gomez W. Bilateral avascular necrosis of the first metatarsal head in adolescence. A case report. Clin Orthop Relat Res 1989;246:282–4.
51. Suzuki J, Tanaka Y, Omokawa S, et al. Idiopathic osteonecrosis of the first metatarsal head: a case report. Clin Orthop Relat Res 2003;415(415):239–43.
52. Monteagudo M, Martínez-de-Albornoz P. Management of complications after hallux valgus reconstruction. Foot Ankle Clin 2020;25(1):151–67.
53. Murdoch DP, Armstrong DG, Dacus JB, et al. The natural history of great toe amputations. J Foot Ankle Surg 1997;36(3):204–56.
54. Hsieh PH, Chang YH, Chen SH, et al. High concentration and bioactivity of vancomycin and aztreonam eluted from Simplex cement spacers in two-stage revision of infected hip implants: a study of 46 patients at an average follow-up of 107 days. J Orthop Res 2006;24(8):1615–21.
55. Myerson MS, Miller SD, Henderson MR, et al. Staged arthrodesis for salvage of the septic hallux metatarsophalangeal joint. Clin Orthop Relat Res 1994;307:174–81.
56. Melamed EA, Peled E. Antibiotic impregnated cement spacer for salvage of diabetic osteomyelitis. Foot Ankle Int 2012;33(3):213–9.

Lisfranc Arthrodesis in Posttraumatic Chronic Injuries

Stefan Rammelt, MD, PhD*, Pablo Andrés Cárdenas Murillo, MD

KEYWORDS

- Midfoot • Tarsometatarsal • Naviculocuneiform • Fracture-dislocation • Arthrosis
- Instability • Deformity • Correction • Interposition Arthroplasty

KEY POINTS

- Subtle injuries and fracture-dislocations at the tarsometatarsal joint if not recognized or treated appropriately result in painful malunions ranging from isolated instability to complex three-dimensional deformities with rapid development of posttraumatic arthritis.
- Deformity correction and fusion of the symptomatic joints leads to significant pain reduction and functional improvement provided that realignment of the anatomic axes is achieved.
- Arthrodesis should be limited to the first to third tarsometatarsal joints whenever possible to preserve flexibility to the lateral foot column. For symptomatic arthritis of the fourth to fifth tarsometatarsal joints interposition arthroplasty is a viable option.
- For complex deformities and instability at the midfoot, corrective fusion is extended to the intercuneiform and naviculocuneiform joints depending on the individual pathology.

INTRODUCTION

Injuries to the tarsometatarsal (TMT; Lisfranc) joint complex are overlooked or underestimated at first presentation with respect to their extent, ligamentous instability, and possible sequelae in 31% to 44% of cases requiring late correction and fusion.[1–7] The reasons for that are manifold and include the low prevalence a great variability of these injuries and a high percentage of multiply injured and polytraumatized patients.[7–10] At initial presentation, subtle clinical and radiographic signs, such as plantar ecchymosis,[11] the linked toe dislocation,[12] and the fleck sign at the base of the second metatarsal,[1] may not be detected. In the absence of adequate radiographs and computed tomography (CT) imaging, unstable Lisfranc injuries may be underestimated and misjudged as "midfoot sprain" or "isolated metatarsal base fracture."[4–7] In particular, subtle Lisfranc injuries with isolated injury to the so-called "Lisfranc ligament" between the first cuneiform and the second metatarsal base, may easily be overlooked if there is no frank diastasis between these bones.[3,13]

University Center for Orthopaedics, Trauma and Plastic Surgery, University Hospital Carl-Gustav Carus at TU Dresden, Fetscherstrasse 74, Dresden 01307, Germany
* Corresponding author.
E-mail address: strammelt@hotmail.com

Foot Ankle Clin N Am 27 (2022) 745–767
https://doi.org/10.1016/j.fcl.2022.07.002
1083-7515/22/© 2022 Elsevier Inc. All rights reserved.

foot.theclinics.com

Another frequent reason for painful posttraumatic deformity and/or instability at the TMT joint with posttraumatic arthritis is inadequate treatment at the time of initial presentation (**Fig. 1**). There is evidence from numerous studies that attempts on closed reduction and cast application or percutaneous K-wire fixation regularly fail to achieve anatomic reduction and thus healing in an adequate position.[1,2,8,9,14] This article reviews the pathoanatomy and correction of posttraumatic Lisfranc joint deformities.

ANATOMY OF THE LISFRANC JOINT COMPLEX

The Lisfranc joint complex is composed of the first to fifth TMT, the four intermetatarsal, and three intertarsal (first and second intercuneiform and the cuneocuboid) joints together with its ligamentous attachments.[15,16] The eponym refers to Jean-Jacques Lisfranc, a Paris-based surgeon of the Napoleonic era, who described in detail the technique of amputation along the TMT joints.[17] The cuneiform bones and the metatarsal bases display a wedge-shaped configuration in the coronal plane, forming a "Roman arch" with the second metatarsal base as the key stone. The latter is indented between the first (medial) and third (lateral) cuneiform, making it prone to fractures with any dislocation at the Lisfranc joint. The mobility of the individual TMT joints varies considerably, with the first, fourth, and fifth being the most mobile and the second and third being the most rigid.[18,19] Biomechanically, the Lisfranc joint complex has been likened to a child's bicycle with the central (second and third) rays being the stable, central wheel and the medial (first) and lateral (fourth and fifth) rays being the supporting wheels at the sides,[20] which is also reflected by a recent classification system of acute Lisfranc injury.[21]

Besides its vault-like bony configuration, the Lisfranc joint complex is stabilized by weak dorsal and strong interosseous and plantar TMT, intermetatarsal, and intertarsal

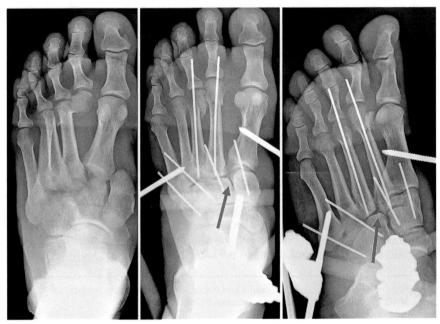

Fig. 1. Limited open reduction and K-wire fixation of a homolateral Lisfranc fracture-dislocation in a 63-year-old male patient. Note the less than optimal reduction of the second and third tarsometatarsal joints with lateral shift of the respective metatarsal bases (*red arrow* in the dorsoplantar radiograph [*middle*] and oblique radiograph [*right*], respectively).

ligaments.[16,22,23] The soft spot for ligamentous injuries is the space between the first and second TMT joints because there is no ligamentous connection between the first and second metatarsal base. The connection between the first cuneiform and the second metatarsal base consists of the Lisfranc ligament.[24] Like the other ligaments in that area it has a dorsal, interosseous, and plantar portion, the latter extending to the third metatarsal base[16,22] A lateral Lisfranc ligament, as described under various names by several anatomists in the 19th century [22] has recently gained renewed attention as it supports the transverse metatarsal arch.[25] It runs plantar from the fifth to the second metatarsal base and blends with the long plantar ligament. The plantar attachments of the tibialis anterior and peroneus longus tendons provide a dynamic support (stirrup) to the TMT joints.[26]

PATHOANATOMY OF POSTTRAUMATIC DEFORMITIES

Overlooked or improperly treated Lisfranc injuries almost invariably result in painful malunion, nonunion, or chronic instability with severely restricted global foot function and rapid progression to posttraumatic arthritis at the Lisfranc joint complex.[1–9,27–29] This applies to subtle Lisfranc injuries and complex TMT fracture-dislocations. Consequently, depending on the nature of the primary injury, a broad spectrum of deformities may be observed.[30]

Overlooked subtle injuries with isolated rupture or avulsion of the Lisfranc ligament lead to chronic instability with progressive planovalgus deformity.[3,4,31,32] In a biomechanical study, simulated dorsolateral dislocation of the second metatarsal base of 2 mm resulted in a 35.5% reduction of the contact surface in the second TMT joint potentially promoting arthritic changes.[33] Furthermore, the frequent avulsion fractures at the second metatarsal base may lead to posttraumatic arthritis. Homolateral fracture-dislocation with lateral deviation of either all or the second to fifth metatarsals with respect to the midfoot results in a fixed forefoot abduction.[34] This subsequently leads to dorsolateral subluxation of the talonavicular and subtalar joints with development of a posttraumatic planovalgus deformity.[2,4,5,35,36]

However, malunion following an axial trauma mechanism leads to cavus or cavovarus deformity with forefoot adduction following insufficiency of the weak dorsal TMT ligaments with consecutive plantarflexion of one or more metatarsals.[2,30,37] This results in overload of the forefoot and metatarsalgia.[31] Divergent and crush injuries to the Lisfranc joint result in complex deformities.

PREOPERATIVE EVALUATION AND PLANNING

Reconstruction of posttraumatic foot and ankle deformities requires a thorough preoperative analysis of the whole lower limb including the previously uninjured side.[30] Because of the thin soft tissue cover over the dorsum of the foot, deformities at the TMT joint are obvious on inspection (**Fig. 2**). The affected foot is examined for scars and callosities. The ankle, subtalar, and midtarsal joints are examined for range of motion, crepitus, and stability. In the TMT joints, local tenderness and sagittal mobility are checked. Rigid plantar flexion of the first metatarsal can cause forefoot-driven hindfoot varus, whereas a hypermobile first metatarsal allows the arch to sink and the hindfoot to go into secondary valgus. The overall foot configuration has to be compared with the unaffected, asymptomatic side (**Fig. 3**). Both feet are evaluated for adequate circulation and sensation and muscle power and balance. The calf is checked for gastrocnemius tightness.[38]

Radiographic evaluation includes standing radiographs in dorsoplantar (anteroposterior) and lateral projections and nonweightbearing oblique (45°) projections for both

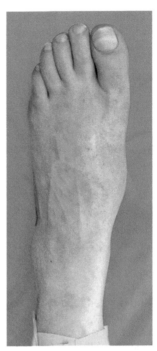

Fig. 2. Clinical aspect of a Lisfranc malunion with obvious abduction of the forefoot and chronic edema over the tarsometatarsal joint.

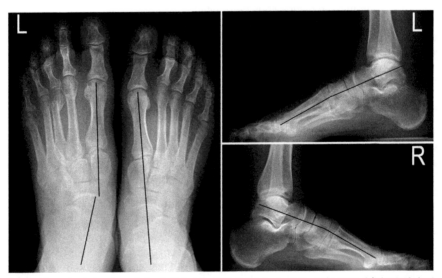

Fig. 3. Chronic abduction of the left forefoot in the tarsometatarsal joint with lateral deviation of the talus–first metatarsal axis in the dorsoplantar view 3 years after the injury (same patient as in **Fig. 1**). In the lateral view the medial arch is less pronounced than on the uninjured right side where the patient has a subtle cavus.

feet (see **Fig. 3**). The images are inspected for any deviations of the talus–first meta-tarsal axis (Meary line) in both planes.[39] Malunited bony avulsions at the base of the second metatarsal may appear as a patchy inhomogeneity (fleck sign) at the base of the second metatarsal.[40] In the dorsoplantar view, the distance between the first and second metatarsal base and malalignment of the lateral border of the second metatarsal with the corresponding edge of the second (middle) cuneiform are checked. Alignment of the third and fourth metatarsal bases with the lateral cuneiform and the cuboid can be best assessed in the 45° oblique view.

CT scanning is helpful in revealing the three-dimensional outline of complex mal-unions, to determine the extent of nonunion, arthritis, avascular necrosis, or bony sequestration in chronic osteitis. It is therefore highly recommended for individual planning of the correction (**Fig. 4**). Weightbearing CT combines the information of standing radiographs and CT scanning and reveals dynamic instabilities. Technetium bone scan or single-photon emission CT/CT is recommended in any case of discrep-ancy between clinical signs and radiographic evidence of arthritis in the single joints (**Fig. 5**).

INDICATIONS FOR ARTHRODESIS AT THE LISFRANC JOINT

In general, arthrodesis should be confined to the symptomatic, arthritic joints as deter-mined with clinical and radiographic analysis of the deformity. A highly unstable first

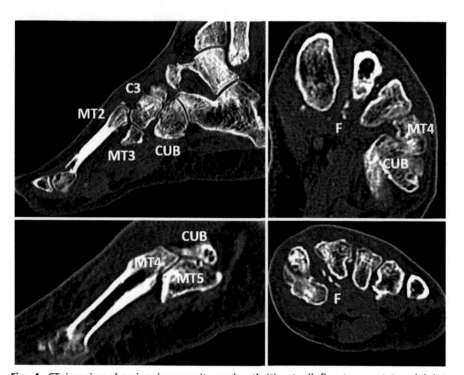

Fig. 4. CT imaging showing incongruity and arthritis at all five tarsometatarsal joints including the fourth and fifth with dorsolateral displacement of the second and third meta-tarsal bases with respect to the corresponding cuneiforms (C3 is shown in the *upper left*), chronic avulsions of the plantar Lisfranc ligament (F in *right*). C, cuneiform; CUB, cuboid; F, chronic fleck sign; MT, metatarsal base. Same patient as in **Figs. 1** and **3**.

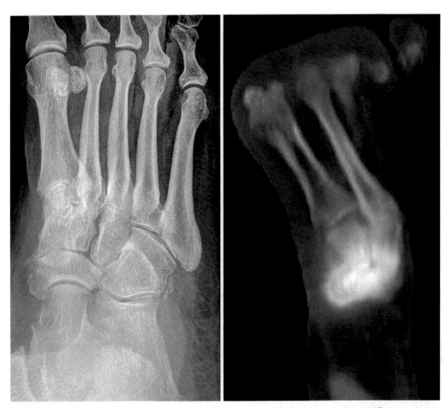

Fig. 5. Single-photon emission CT/CT of a patient with diffuse pain in the midfoot and signs of arthritis in the tarsometatarsal and naviculocuneiform joints on the oblique radiograph (*left*). Single-photon emission CT/CT reveals active arthritis at the medial and intermediate (first and second) naviculocuneiform joints but not the tarsometatarsal joints. This patient needs a naviculocuneiform rather than a tarsometatarsal fusion.

TMT joint should be included generously into the fusion because a hypermobile first metatarsal may contribute to TMT deformity and arthritis.[30,38] In addition, patients experience virtually no functional loss after fusion of the first to third TMT joints, whereas the fourth and fifth TMT joints, which have a considerable amount of sagittal motion essential for normal gait,[41] usually are not as susceptible to arthritis but fusion of these joints regularly results in a stiff lateral column with functional restrictions and lateral-sided pain.[2,30,36,38]

Deformity correction is achieved with asymmetric resection of the TMT joints. In case of avascular necrosis or loss of length of a single ray, autologous bone grafting is used.[5,36] In selected patients with a high demand on a flexible midfoot, such as elite gymnasts and dancers, ligamentoplasty with tendon graft or flexible implant has been described as a viable alternative to fusion for chronic instability following rupture of the Lisfranc ligament.[32,42,43]

SURGICAL TECHNIQUE
Corrective Fusion of the First to Third Tarsometatarsal Joint

The patient is positioned supine on the operating table with a wedge-shaped support under the ipsilateral hip so that the affected foot rests with the toes pointing nearly straight up. The exact position and number of dorsal incisions depends on the individual pathology. For correction and fusion of the first to third TMT joints, a longitudinal medial incision is centered over the second metatarsal. For isolated pathologies at the first and second TMT joint including chronic rupture of the Lisfranc ligament, the incision is made in the interval between the two. To address the lateral TMT joints, a second incision is made parallel to the first one in the space between the fourth and fifth metatarsals and extends up and over the cuboid.

Correction starts at the second metatarsal base, which is the apex of the deformity in most cases. It is considered the keystone and thus the key to reduction of the TMT joints.[5,30] The space between the second metatarsal and the medial cuneiform is cleared from remaining bony debris and fibrous tissue. The first to third TMT joints are cleared from residual cartilage and are excised in a wedge-like manner to correct any abduction/adduction and dorsiflexion/plantarflexion..

In many instances, the fourth and fifth metatarsals are brought into anatomic alignment to the cuboid bone once realignment of the medial column had been accomplished.[6] If this is not the case, the fourth and fifth cuboid-metatarsal joints are visualized through the lateral incision between the two. In cases of long-standing arthrosis, spurs or hypertrophic bone have to be excised with an osteotome to get a clear view of the remaining joints.[30] The joints are then freed from adhesions and inspected for remaining cartilage and mobilized.

Following debridement and mobilization, the TMT joints are brought into correct alignment and apposition in transverse (abduction/adduction) and sagittal (plantar flexion-dorsiflexion) planes. Usually, the relative length of the metatarsals is corrected by shortening the second and possibly third metatarsal bases. In case of substantial traumatic bone loss because of necrosis, correct length is obtained with autologous bone graft. Depending on the size of the defect, either structural bicortical grafts or loose cancellous bone chips are used, mostly from the ipsilateral crest.

Particular care is taken to realign the second metatarsal base to all three surfaces: (1) the debrided lateral wall of the first cuneiform, (2) the debrided distal joint surface of the second cuneiform, and (3) toward the medial aspect of the third cuneiform. A pointed reduction clamp between the medial cortex of the first cuneiform and the lateral cortex of the second or third metatarsal base is most helpful for that (**Fig. 6**). The notch where the base of the second metatarsal is reduced anatomically must be without any remaining gap or shift. The second TMT joint is held temporarily with a retrograde Kirschner wire. Then, the first and third metatarsals are realigned to the second TMT joint and transfixed with K-wires. For placement of the wires, the surgeon must hold the alignment securely while keeping the metatarsal heads level to avoid any residual sagittal deformity.

The first screw (a 3.5- or 4.0-mm cortical screw) is routinely placed along the same direction as the reduction clamp through a stab wound at an angle of approximately 45 degrees from the medial side of the first cuneiform into the base of the second metatarsal, lagging the base of the second metatarsal compactly into this notch (see **Fig. 6**). This screw replaces the dysfunctional Lisfranc ligament. The second 3.5- or 4.0-mm cortical screw is inserted through a countersunk hole or trough made 2 cm distal to the joint on the cortical dorsum of the first metatarsal (**Fig. 7**). The third and fourth screws are usually started from the dorsolateral second and third metatarsals. They are aimed proximally and medially and inserted into the second and third cuneiforms, respectively. The screw in the third TMT joint is inserted through a stab incision. After each metatarsal-cuneiform joint is stabilized, the accuracy of its position and alignment is verified clinically and fluoroscopically. If believed necessary, a second (2.7-mm or 3.5-mm) screw may be added across each joint, usually going from proximal

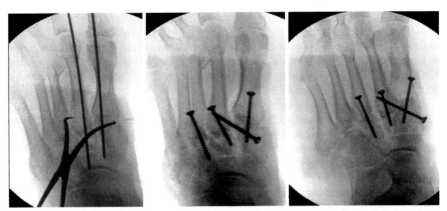

Fig. 6. Stepwise correction of a chronic homolateral Lisfranc injury following debridement and mobilization. Reduction starts with the second metatarsal base and fusion is confined to the first to third tarsometatarsal joints. Same patient as in **Figs. 1, 3,** and **4.**

to distal. The second screw may be smaller because its purpose is to control rotation, not provide leverage for holding power. In analogy, a neutralization screw may be placed upward and laterally from the plantar metaphysis of the first metatarsal into the second cuneiform. With gross intercuneiform instability, an additional screw may be placed via stab incisions from medial to lateral.

Management of Fourth/Fifth Tarsometatarsal Joint Arthritis and Deformity

There are no clear recommendations for the treatment of arthrosis in the fourth and fifth TMT joints. These joints frequently remain symptomatic after fusion because the amount of motion they normally have is needed to provide cushioning along the

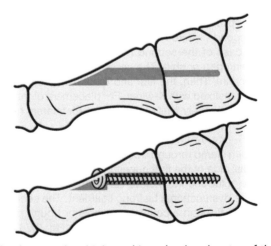

Fig. 7. A trough for the screw head is burred into the dorsal cortex of the first metatarsal, ideally about 2.0 cm distal to the joint. Next, a 3.5- or 4.0-mm gliding hole is drilled into the base of the metatarsal, and a 2.5-mm tap hole is drilled into the first cuneiform. (*From* Rammelt S, Zwipp H, Hansen ST. Posttraumatic reconstruction of the foot and ankle. In: Browner BD, Jupiter JB, Krettek C, Anderson PA (eds.): Skeletal Trauma, 6th Edition, Philadelphia, Elsevier Saunders, 2019, pp 2641-2690.)

lateral border of the foot.[38] Including them into the fusion of the Lisfranc joints has been associated with significantly inferior results than isolated fusion of the medial (first to third) TMT joints.[2,28,36]

If nonoperative management including physical therapy, the use of orthotics, or a thick, soft-soled shoe fails to alleviate the symptoms, dorsal cheilectomy provides pain relief and increased motion in less severe cases.[30] Other options include simple resection arthroplasty and interposition of local fascia, tendon, spherical or biconcave ceramic or polymeric implants,[30,44,45] but reports on either of these methods are scarce and there is no definitive solution to cuboid fourth and fifth metatarsal joint arthrosis. In the authors' experience, debridement and interposition arthroplasty with the peroneus tertius tendon (**Fig. 8**) has been successful in relieving symptoms while preserving some elasticity to the lateral foot column (**Fig. 9**).

Correction of Complex Deformities

In the presence of traumatic arthrosis of the naviculocuneiform joint and/or a sag or a break in the talar–first metatarsal axis at this level (**Fig. 10**), the naviculocuneiform has to be realigned and fused. This is achieved with crossed screws that are advanced from the medial cuneiform into the lateral navicular and vice versa. Alternatively, staples or plates may be used as fixation in this area (**Fig. 11**). After fixation, cancellous autograft may be added to enhance bone healing. The bone chips are typically used to fill remaining gaps after debridement of the joints. Alternatively, divots are burred across the dorsal aspect of each joint and are filled with cancellous bone chips.[38]

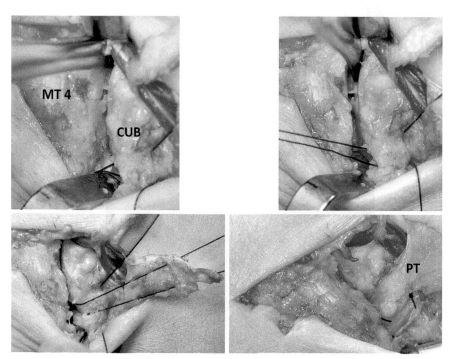

Fig. 8. Interposition arthroplasty following debridement and realignment of the arthritic fourth and fifth tarsometatarsal joints with the peroneus tertius (PT) tendon that is fixed into the resected joint with transosseous sutures between the fourth metatarsal base (MT 4) and the cuboid (CUB). Same patient as in **Figs. 1, 3, 4,** and **6**.

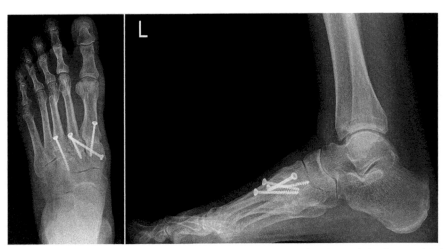

Fig. 9. Standing radiographs at 1 year following corrective arthrodesis of the first to third tarsometatarsal joint and interposition arthroplasty of the fourth and fifth tarsometatarsal joint showing a stable, plantigrade foot with anatomic alignment. Same patient as in **Figs. 1, 3, 4, 6,** and **8.**

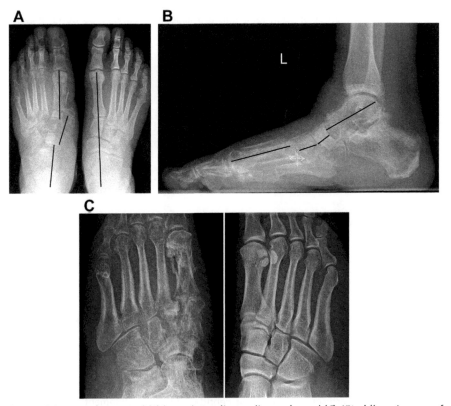

Fig. 10. (A) Dorsoplantar and (B) lateral standing radiographs and (C) 45° oblique images of a patient with complex (multilevel) posttraumatic deformity of the midfoot 7 months following crush injury to the midfoot in a 47-year-old male patient.

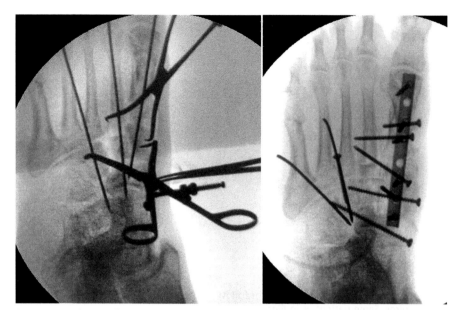

Fig. 11. Correction of the medial column following debridement and temporary fixation with reduction clamps and K-wires. Fusion of the first to third tarsometatarsal and naviculocuneiform joints is achieved with screws. In addition, because of the complex deformity, a dorsal bridge plate was applied from the first metatarsal to the navicular leaving the essential talonavicular joint free. Same patient as in **Fig. 10**.

The graft may be cancellous bone that was removed in the course of shaping the joints, usually from osteophytes. If this amount of bone is inadequate, particularly if necrotic or sclerotic bone had to be removed, more cancellous bone may be harvested from the lateral calcaneus or distal tibial metaphysis. At the end of the procedure, dorsoplantar (anteroposterior), lateral, and 45° oblique radiographs are taken with simulated loading and the foot in a neutral position to verify the position of the implants and realignment of the midfoot and forefoot.

Note that a tight gastrocnemius aggravates stress across the midfoot.[30,38] If the surgeon decides to carry out a gastrocnemius slide after examining the patient's contralateral foot, it is done after fusing the Lisfranc joint. A gastrocnemius release should be considered whenever a patient cannot move the foot easily to 10° or 15° of dorsiflexion with the knee straight during at preoperative examination (Silfverskiöld test).

Postoperative Management

The lower leg and foot are immobilized with a splint and elevated for 2 or 3 days. Range of motion exercises of the ankle and subtalar joint are initiated. After the initial swelling has subsided, the patient is allowed to ambulate on crutches with weight-of-leg weightbearing (20 kg) in a removable, individually molded cast shoe[46] that leaves the ankle mobile but avoids any forefoot push-off for 8 to 12 weeks. The exact time of protection depends on the individual bone quality, extent of arthrodesis, type of fixation, and necessity of bone grafting. Weightbearing is gradually increased after union has been demonstrated in standing radiographs (**Fig. 12**). It may take 3 to 6 months before swelling and discomfort completely resolve (**Fig. 13**). Physical therapy aims at regaining muscle strength and a normal gait pattern and maintaining range of

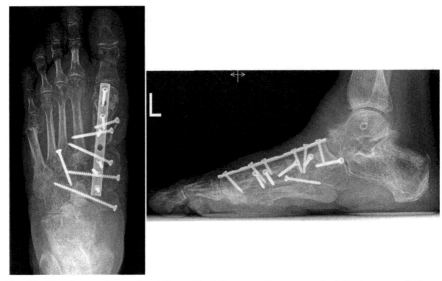

Fig. 12. Standing radiographs at 6-months follow-up after removal of the temporarily introduced K-wires. Same patient as in **Figs. 10** and **11**.

motion at the ankle, subtalar, and midtarsal joints, which together with the fourth and fifth TMT joints will preserve all essential motion at the foot even after extended Lisfranc fusion (**Fig. 14**). Implants need only be removed if symptomatic. Because the foot is less flexible following TMT fusion, a shoe with a thick cushioning fixed sole and soft accommodative orthoses may be applied.

COMPLICATIONS

The reported complication rates following TMT fusion vary considerably in the available literature because of different reported causes and techniques. Wound healing problems including superficial infection and wound slough are reported in 3% to 10% of cases,[5,28,47–49] and deep infections in 1% to 4%.[28,49,50] Although the former typically heal with local wound care and antiseptic dressings, the latter frequently require surgical revision.

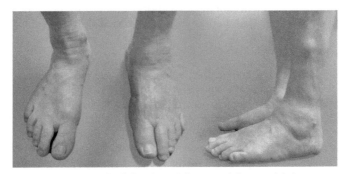

Fig. 13. Clinical images 6 months following Lisfranc and first to third tarsometatarsal and naviculocuneiform arthrodesis showing a stable, plantigrade foot. Same patient as in **Figs. 10–12**.

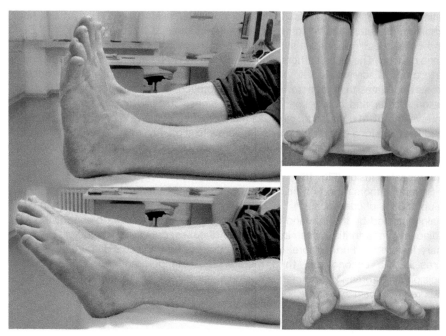

Fig. 14. Range of motion at 6 months showing only marginallylimited range of motion despite extensile fusion. Same patient as in **Figs. 10–13**.

Nonunion is a typical complication after fusion (**Fig. 15**). It may affect one or more TMT joints and is not always symptomatic.[2,5,28] Reported union rates following TMT joint fusion for posttraumatic deformity correction range from 81% to 100%.[2,6,28,47–51] The rates are similar for isolated second TMT fusion,[52] midfoot, and hindfoot fusions using

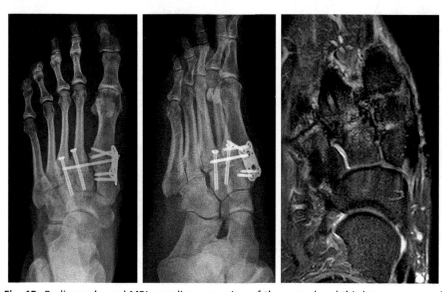

Fig. 15. Radiographs and MRI revealing nonunion of the second and third tarsometatarsal joints after attempted fusion of the first to third tarsometatarsal joints with cannulated 3.5-mm screws and a medial plate.

Nitinol staples.[53] Reported risk factors for nonunion include a high body mass index, smoking, diabetes, and a high number of fused joints at the same foot.[48,50,54] Buda and colleagues[50] reported a significantly decreased risk of nonunion with the use of bone grafting. The same authors found plate fixation to be at a higher risk for nonunion than crossed screws (16.4% vs 4.8%). Ettinger et al.[48] found higher fusion rates for srews and plates than for screws only. In a biomechanical cadaver model of first TMT fusion, Baxter and colleagues[55] showed a higher stability for crossed screws over screws and plate constructs, whereas Marks and colleagues[56] demonstrated a higher load to failure for a plantar plate than for screw fixation. Aiyer and colleagues[57] found a superiority for Nitinol staples. Symptomatic nonunions require surgical revision with debridement of the pseudoarthrosis, drilling of the subcortical bone, bone grafting, and repeated fusion (**Fig. 16**).

Several authors report on prominent or loose hardware requiring a second surgery in up to 39% of cases.[27,47,49,50,58] This seems to be independent of the implants and mainly caused by the thin and delicate soft tissue cover of the dorsum of the foot. Adjacent joint arthritis is seen in up to 10% of cases, depending on the extent of primary fusion.[48,49] Furthermore, less frequent reported complications are stress fractures at the second and third metatarsals,[34] tendon adhesions,[47] neuritis or incisional neuroma,[28,34] metatarsalgia and sesamoiditis,[48,59] malunion,[36,57] and complex regional pain syndrome.[28]

OUTCOMES

Numerous prospective studies have shown that corrective arthrodesis of the Lisfranc joint results in a significant reduction of pain and improvement of foot function after initially overlooked or improperly treated Lisfranc fracture dislocations.[2,6,28] The

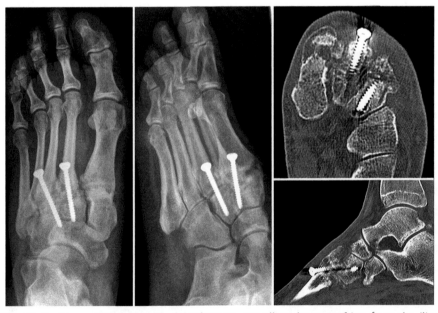

Fig. 16. Revision arthrodesis with debridement, cancellous bone grafting from the iliac crest, and solid 4.0-mm screws was carried out (*left*). CT scan at 6 months postoperatively demonstrates solid union (*right*). Same patient as in **Fig. 15**.

main results from clinical studies on corrective Lisfranc fusion since 1990 are provided in **Table 1**. When reviewing the pertinent literature, it becomes apparent that only a few studies deal exclusively with posttraumatic arthritis and deformities, whereas most report the results of Lisfranc fusion for various etiologies including degenerative, rheumatic, and other inflammatory arthritis. A large body of literature deals with fusion of the first TMT joint for correction of hallux valgus with hypermobile first ray and primary medial Lisfranc joint fusion for acute ligamentous injuries. Both are beyond the scope of this review.

The existing studies on corrective arthrodesis for chronic injury unanimously report high rates of patient satisfaction and good to excellent results in 69% to 93% of cases using different scoring systems. Alignment of the anatomic axes, when reported, was significantly improved,[6,27,28,48,50] which is an important prerequisite for obtaining good results. If this is achieved, the loss of motion from fusing the first to third TMT joints is well tolerated by the patients.[30] However, several authors reported adjacent degenerative joint arthritis in 10% to 16%.[48,49] The latter seems to be related to the number of joints fused.

In one study comparing primary open reduction and internal fixation of TMT fracture-dislocations with secondary arthrodesis for posttraumatic malunions at an average of 22 months postinjury, primary open reduction and internal fixation gave significantly better functional results after 3 years follow-up and earlier return to work than secondary arthrodesis.[6] The authors concluded that long-standing deformities lead to soft tissue contractions and warranted extensive exposure of the joints and sometimes bone grafting thus resulting in a greater amount of scarring in the secondary treatment group. The high satisfaction rate (90%) in the arthrodesis group despite the inferior functional results may be attributed to the relief of pain and highly significant functional improvement compared with the preoperative state. Complex Lisfranc injuries with severe bony comminution and soft tissue damage regularly need staged treatment with early fusion in combination with free microvascular flap coverage to obtain a stable, plantigrade foot with durable soft tissue cover.[7,60,61] The debate of primary fusion versus internal fixation for acute purely ligamentous Lisfranc injuries is beyond the topic of this review.

Several authors have suggested that inclusion of the fourth and fifth TMT joints into the fusion may result in inferior outcomes than fusion of the first to third TMT joints only,[2,28,38] which is supported by the findings of Lin and colleagues[36] who found significantly lower scores after fusion of the fourth and fifth TMT joints. This is explained by the higher mobility in these joints.[19,41] However, some improvement in pain scores has been reported in one study after isolated fusion of the lateral (fourth to fifth) TMT joints for severe arthritis.[62] In the authors' practice, fusion is generally limited to the medial column and in case of lateral arthritis, an interposition arthroplasty is preferred (see **Figs. 6–9**). However, data on outcome of any procedure for fourth and fifth TMT are scarce.

Further negative prognostic factors include long delay between trauma and correction,[2] eligibility for workers' compensation,[36] a body mass index greater than 30,[50] smoking, and a higher number of fused joints.[48,54] Return to work is achieved by 67% to 98% of patients[47,63] depending on their individual demands, but patients should be counseled that only about half of them will be able to perform all preinjury activities including sports.[58]

In summary, corrective arthrodesis provides significant relief of pain and functional rehabilitation in patients with painful malunions following Lisfranc injuries. However, a full return to all preinjury activities cannot be guaranteed. The focus must be on

Table 1
Main results from clinical studies dealing with corrective fusion of the Lisfranc joint for posttraumatic and other deformities since 1990

First Author (Year)	Cases	Follow-up	Technique	Complications	Union Rate (%)	Main Results
Sangeorzan (1990)	16	28 mo	Lag screws; Bone-grafting not necessary for most patients	1 nonunion requiring revision	94	69% good to excellent results; Long delay and work-related accidents were negative prognostic factors
Horton (1993)	9	27 mo	1/3 tubular medial plate; 6 deformity corrections; 3 in situ fusions	1 prominent plate; 1 screw loosening	100	Fusion within 12 weeks all improved, 7/9 good to excellent results; Lateral TFMA improved an average of 15.5° and AP TFMA 10° after deformity correction
Komenda (1996)	32	50 mo	Cancellous/cortical screws; 24 autogenous bone grafts; 8 claw-toe corrections; 3 posterior tibial tendon reconstructions; 3 interdigital neuroma resections	3 neuritis; 2 metatarsalgia; 2 malunion; 1 wound slough, superficial infection, and CRPS	97	AOFAS midfoot score improved from 44 to 78 ($P = 0.02$); Correction of AP TFMA (from 13° to 0°), lateral TFMA (from 16° to 4°), 4° of residual abduction
Mann (1996)	41	6 y	17 interfragmentary screws; 15 plate and screws; 5 staples, 4 other; 11 bone grafts (for posttraumatic, degenerative, inflammatory midtarsal and TMT arthritis)	2 skin slough; 3 stress fractures of the second metatarsal; 3 incisional neuroma	98	38 of 41 feet (93%) with satisfactory result realignment of the midfoot was achieved; Interfragmentary screws or a medial plate, or both preferred
Treadwell (1998)	9	29 mo	Cannulated cancellous self-tapping partially threaded screws for chronic injury	1 asymptomatic nonunion of first TMT joint	89	Good results in 78%; Fair and poor results in 11% each

Study	N	Follow-up	Procedure	Complications		Outcomes
Lin (2000)	16	36 mo	Iliac crest bone grafting and K-wire fixation for posttraumatic or primary degenerative disease	1 nonunion 1 delayed union 1 varus malunion	94	AOFAS improved by 41 points FFI decreased from 64 to 24 81% rated results as good to excellent 75% returned to previous level of activity Fusion of the fourth and fifth TMT joints and workers' compensation claims associated with poorer outcomes radiographic parameters significantly improved
Rammelt (2008)	20	36 mo	Screws, plates for posttraumatic arthritis and malunion, fusion of the first to third TMT joint only in 14 cases	One soft tissue infection (5%) One symptomatic nonunion (5%) No deep infections	90	Significant improvement of AOFAS score (17.9–71.8) Significant higher score in a control group of 20 patients with primary ORIF (81.4) Radiographic parameters close to physiologic values
Nemec (2011)	74	56 mo	Primary midfoot arthritis with deformity (collapse) 87% gastrocnemius contracture	3 deep infections 1 CRPS 11 reoperations in addition to 26 symptomatic hardware removals	92	Significant improvement in the TFMA and medial cuneiform height Pain improved from 7 to 2 (VAS) AOFAS score improved from 32 to 79 90% patient satisfaction BMI >30 associated with poorer outcomes and nonunion
Filippi (2012)	72	NS	Hybrid fixation technique (plate with locked and lag screws) for primary and posttraumatic arthritis, instability, nonunion	4% wound dehiscence 6% neuropraxia 3% hardware irritation 3% tendon adhesion	93	Time to union 6–16 weeks 71/72 return to preinjury activities between 0 and 12 months

(continued on next page)

Table 1
(continued)

First Author (Year)	Cases	Follow-up	Technique	Complications	Union Rate (%)	Main Results
Gougoulias (2016)	30	24 mo	12 screws/18 plates and screws for degenerative, rheumatic, and posttraumatic arthritis 3 gastrocnemius releases	16.6% complications 20% unplanned reoperations No wound complications	93	47% excellent, 43% good, 10% fair/poor Time to union 12.9 weeks All had a plantigrade foot, 30% had residual pain in adjacent joints 67% returned to full-time employment
Buda (2018)	88	78 mo	Screws (55.6%), plates (35.5%), hybrid fixation (9%), bone grafting (79.6%)	3.4% delayed wound healing 1.1% deep infection 15.9% painful hardware 3.4% hardware loosening 10.2% adjacent joint arthritis 35.2% reoperations	89	Nonunion associated with (1) arthrodesis using plate fixation with all screws through the plate, (2) smoking, and (3) postoperative nonanatomic alignment Bone grafting significantly lowered the nonunion rate Delayed wound healing after plate fixation only Association between complication rate and number of columns fused
Saxena (2021)	187	2.4 y	3.5-mm screws across the joints or plates spanning the joints with 2.7- to 3.5-mm screws 133 (70.7%) with chronic injury 55 (29.3%) with acute injury 48% gastrocnemius recession (38% midtarsal and subtalar fusions)	16% secondary degenerative arthrosis 39% symptomatic hardware removal 4% malunion	81	Return to activity after approximately 3 mo 59% return to activity including sports 27% could not return to impact sports Highest nonunion rate for NC and TN fusion

| Ettinger (2021) | 103 | 47 mo | Crossed screws and/or locking plate fixation for arthritis/deformities of multiple causes | 11% metatarsalgia 10% wound healing disorders 4% secondary degenerative changes and sesamoid arthritis 25% overall reoperation rate | 87 | All scores (EFAS, FAOS, NRS, SF-36) improved significantly except for the UCLA score All radiologic measurements improved significantly Return to work at 6 weeks, sports at 22 weeks Less nonunions with plate and screw fixation compared with crossed screws only BMI >27 and smoking were associated with nonunion and wound healing problems Arthritis of more than 2 columns leads to inferior results |

Studies on fusion of a single TMT joint (mostly first and second), on in situ fusion for purely degenerative arthritis, on primary fusion for acute trauma only, and studies on fusion for Charcot neuropathy were excluded.

Abbreviations: AOFAS, American Orthopaedic Foot and Ankle Society; AP, anteroposterior; BMI, body mass index; CRPS, complex regional pain syndrome; EFAS, European Society for Foot and Ankle Surgery; FAOS, Foot and Ankle Outcome Score; FFI, Foot Function Index; NC, naviculocuneiform; NRS, Numeric Rating Scale; NS, not stated; ORIF, open reduction and internal fixation; SF-36, Short Form-36; TFMA, talus–first metatarsal angle; TN, talonavicular; VAS, Visual Analogue Scale.

detecting the sometimes subtle clinical and radiographic signs of these injuries and adequate reduction and stabilization in the first place to avoid long-standing deformities.

CLINICS CARE POINTS

- Care must be taken to ensure proper evaluation and treatment of subtle injuries and fracture-dislocations at the tarsometatarsal joint at first presentation to avoid painful malunion, instability, and arthritis.
- Planning of corrective surgery requires a thorough clinical and radiographic assessment of the three-dimensional deformity.
- Correction of malunited Lisfranc injuries includes debridement and fusion of the symptomatic joints with realignment of the talus–first metatarsal axis in the horizontal and sagittal planes.
- For isolated chronic injury to the Lisfranc ligament in professional dancers or athletes, a ligamentoplasty is a good alternative to fusion.
- Arthrodesis should be limited to the first to third tarsometatarsal joints whenever possible to preserve flexibility to the lateral foot column.
- For symptomatic arthritis of the fourth to fifth tarsometatarsal joints, debridement and interposition arthroplasty with fascia, tendon, or ceramic implants have been proposed with scarce evidence in the literature for any single method.
- For complex deformities and instability at the midfoot, the intercuneiform and naviculocuneiform joints should be included into the correction and fusion saving the talonavicular joint whenever possible.
- Corrective arthrodesis reportedly leads to significant pain reduction and functional improvement in chronic Lisfranc injuries.

DISCLOSURE

S. Rammelt is a paid consultant of KLS Martin and 3M. He received travel support and payment for presentations from Siemens Healthineers and AO Trauma. No conflict of interest results with respect to the content of this review article. P. A. Cárdenas Morillo has nothing to disclose.

REFERENCES

1. Myerson MS, Fisher RT, Burgess AR, et al. Fracture dislocations of the tarsometatarsal joints: end results correlated with pathology and treatment. Foot Ankle 1986;6(5):225–42.
2. Sangeorzan BJ, Veith RG, Hansen ST Jr. Salvage of Lisfranc's tarsometatarsal joint by arthrodesis. Foot Ankle 1990;10(4):193–200.
3. Faciszewski T, Burks RT, Manaster BJ. Subtle injuries of the Lisfranc joint. J Bone Joint Surg Am 1990;72(10):1519–22.
4. Petje G, Schiller C, Steinböck G. Mobile flatfoot as a sequela of dislocation injury of the Lisfranc joint. A retrospective analysis of 13 patients. Unfallchirurg 1997;100(10):787–91 [Article in German].
5. Zwipp H, Rammelt S, Holch M, et al. Lisfranc arthrodesis after malunited fracture healing. Unfallchirurg 1999;102(12):918–23 [Article in German].

6. Rammelt S, Schneiders W, Schikore H, et al. Primary open reduction and fixation compared with delayed corrective arthrodesis in the treatment of tarsometatarsal (Lisfranc) fracture-dislocation. J Bone Joint Surg Br 2008;90:1499–506.
7. Rammelt S. Chopart and Lisfranc joint injuries. In: Bentley G, editor. European surgical orthopaedics and traumatology. The EFORT textbook. Berlin, Heidelberg, New York: Springer; 2014. p. 3835–57.
8. Arntz CT, Veith RG, Hansen ST Jr. Fractures and fracture-dislocations of the tarsometatarsal joint. J Bone Joint Surg Am 1988;70(2):173–81.
9. Richter M, Wippermann B, Krettek C, et al. Fractures and fracture dislocations of the midfoot: occurrence, causes and long-term results. Foot Ankle Int 2001;22(5):392–8.
10. Haapamaki V, Kiuru M, Koskinen S. Lisfranc fracture-dislocation in patients with multiple trauma: diagnosis with multidetector computed tomography. Foot Ankle Int 2004;25(9):614–9.
11. Ross G, Cronin R, Hauzenblas J, et al. Plantar ecchymosis sign: a clinical aid to diagnosis of occult Lisfranc tarsometatarsal injuries. J Orthop Trauma 1996;10(2):119–22.
12. English TA. Dislocations of the metatarsal bone and adjacent toe. J Bone Joint Surg Br 1964;46:700–4.
13. Nunley JA, Vertullo CJ. Classification, investigation, and management of midfoot sprains: Lisfranc injuries in the athlete. Am J Sports Med 2002;30(6):871–8.
14. Calder JD, Whitehouse SL, Saxby TS. Results of isolated Lisfranc injuries and the effect of compensation claims. J Bone Joint Surg Br 2004;86(4):527–30.
15. de Palma L, Santucci A, Sabetta SP, et al. Anatomy of the Lisfranc joint complex. Foot Ankle Int 1997;18(6):356–64.
16. Castro M, Melão L, Canella C, et al. Lisfranc joint ligamentous complex: MRI with anatomic correlation in cadavers. AJR Am J Roentgenol 2010;195(6):W447–55.
17. Lisfranc J. Nouvelle methode operatoire pour l'amputation partielle du pied par son articulation tarso-metatarsienne. Paris: L'Imprimerie Feuguery; 1815.
18. Honnart F. Anatomie et physiologie de l'avant-pied. Rev Chir Orthop Reparatrice Appar Mot 1974;60(Suppl 2):107–12.
19. Ouzounian TJ, Shereff MJ. In vitro determination of midfoot motion. Foot Ankle 1989;10:140–6.
20. De Doncker E, Kowalski C. The normal and pathological foot. Concepts of anatomy, physiology and pathology of foot deformities. Acta Orthop Belg 1970;36(4):386–551 [Article in French].
21. Schepers T, Rammelt S. Classifying the Lisfranc injury: literature overview and a new classification. FussSprungg 2018;16:151–9.
22. Fick R. Handbuch der Anatomie und Mechanik der Gelenke unter Berücksichtigung der bewegenden Muskeln. Part I: Anatomie der Gelenke. Jena: Fischer; 1904.
23. Solan MC, Moorman CT 3rd, Miyamoto RG, et al. Ligamentous restraints of the second tarsometatarsal joint: a biomechanical evaluation. Foot Ankle Int 2001;22:637–41.
24. Quenu E, Kuss G. Etude sur les luxations du metatarse (luxations metatarsotarsiennes) du diastasis entre le 1. et le 2. metatarsien. Rev Chir Paris 1909;39:281–336.
25. Mason L, Jayatilaka MLT, Fisher A, et al. Anatomy of the lateral plantar ligaments of the transverse metatarsal. Arch Foot Ankle Int 2020;41(1):109–14.
26. Voss H, Herrlinger R, Taschenbuch der Anatomie. Einführung in die Anatomie, Bewegungsapparat. Band 1. Jena. 17th Ed. Gustav Fischer Verlag; 1983.

27. Horton GA, Olney BW. Deformity correction and arthrodesis of the midfoot with a medial plate. Foot Ankle 1993;14(9):493–9.
28. Komenda GA, Myerson MS, Biddinger KR. Results of arthrodesis of the tarsometatarsal joints after traumatic injury. J Bone Joint Surg Am 1996;78(11):1665–76.
29. Mittlmeier T, Haar P, Beck M. Reconstruction after malunited Lisfranc injuries. Eur J Trauma Emerg Med 2010;36:217–26.
30. Rammelt S, Zwipp H, Hansen ST. Posttraumatic reconstruction of the foot and ankle. In: Browner BD, Jupiter JB, Krettek C, et al, editors. Skeletal trauma. 6th Edition. Philadelphia: Elsevier Saunders; 2019. p. 2641–90.
31. Zwipp H, Rammelt S. Tscherne unfallchirurgie. Fuss. Berlin, Heidelberg, New York: Springer; 2014.
32. Nery C, Raduan F, Baumfeld D. Joint-sparing corrections in malunited Lisfranc joint injuries. Foot Ankle Clin 2016;21(1):161–76.
33. Ebraheim NA, Yang H, Lu J, et al. Computer evaluation of second tarsometatarsal joint dislocation. Foot Ankle Int 1996;17:685–9.
34. Mann RA, Prieskorn D, Sobel M. Mid-tarsal and tarsometatarsal arthrodesis for primary degenerative osteoarthrosis or osteoarthrosis after trauma. J Bone Joint Surg Am 1996;78:1376–85.
35. Brunet JA, Wiley JJ. The late results of tarsometatarsal joint injuries. J Bone Joint Surg Br 1987;69(3):437–40.
36. Lin SS, Bono CM, Treuting R, et al. Limited intertarsal arthrodesis using bone grafting and pin fixation. Foot Ankle Int 2000;21(9):742–8.
37. Rammelt S, Schneiders W, Zwipp H. Corrective tarsometatarsal arthrodesis for malunion after fracture-dislocation. Orthopade 2006;35(4):435–42 [Article in German].
38. Hansen STJ. Functional reconstruction of the foot and ankle. Philadelphia: Williams & Wilkins; 2000.
39. Meary R. Le pied creux essentiel. Rev Chir Orthop Reparatrice Appar Mot 1967; 53(5):389–410.
40. Jeffreys TE. Lisfranc's fracture-dislocation. J Bone Joint Surg Br 1963;45:546–51.
41. Lundgren P, et al. Invasive in vivo measurement of rear-, mid- and forefoot motion during walking. Gait Posture 2008;28(1):93–100.
42. Zwipp H, Rammelt S. Anatomical reconstruction of chronically instable Lisfranc's ligaments. Unfallchirurg 2014;117(9):791–7 [Article in German].
43. Charlton T, Boe C, Thordarson DB. Suture button fixation treatment of chronic Lisfranc injury in professional dancers and high-level athletes. J Dance Med Sci 2015;19(4):135–9.
44. Berlet GC, Hodges Davis W, Anderson RB. Tendon arthroplasty for basal fourth and fifth metatarsal arthritis. Foot Ankle Int 2002;23(5):440–6.
45. Shawen SB, Anderson RB, Cohen BE, et al. Spherical ceramic interpositional arthroplasty for basal fourth and fifth metatarsal arthritis. Foot Ankle Int 2007;28(8):896–901.
46. Rammelt S, Swords M, Dhillon M, et al, editors. Manual of fracture management. Foot & ankle. Stuttgart – New York and Davos: Thieme and AO Foundation; 2020.
47. Filippi J, Myerson MS, Scioli MW, et al. Midfoot arthrodesis following multi-joint stabilization with a novel hybrid plating system. Foot Ankle Int 2012;33(3):220–5.
48. Ettinger S, Altemeier A, Stukenborg-Colsman C, et al. Comparison of isolated screw to plate and screw fixation for tarsometatarsal arthrodesis including clinical outcome predictors. Foot Ankle Int 2021;42(6):734–43.
49. Nemec SA, Habbu RA, Anderson JG, et al. Outcomes following midfoot arthrodesis for primary arthritis. Foot Ankle Int 2011;32(4):355–61.

50. Buda M, Hagemeijer NC, Kink S, et al. Effect of fixation type and bone graft on tarsometatarsal fusion. Foot Ankle Int 2018;39(12):1394–402.
51. Treadwell JR, Kahn MD. Lisfranc arthrodesis for chronic pain: a cannulated screw technique. J Foot Ankle Surg 1998;37(1):28–36.
52. Kilmartin TE, O'Kane C. Fusion of the second metatarsocuneiform joint for the painful osteoarthrosis. Foot Ankle Int 2008;29(11):1079–87.
53. Schipper ON, Ford SE, Moody PW, et al. Radiographic results of nitinol compression staples for hindfoot and midfoot arthrodeses. Foot Ankle Int 2018;39(2): 172–9.
54. Dang DY, Flint WW, Haytmanek CT, et al. Locked dorsal compression plate arthrodesis for degenerative arthritis of the midfoot. J Foot Ankle Surg 2020; 59(6):1171–6.
55. Baxter JR, Mani SB, Chan JY, et al. Crossed-screws provide greater tarsometatarsal fusion stability compared to compression plates. Foot Ankle Spec 2015; 8(2):95–100.
56. Marks RM, Parks BG, Schon LC. Midfoot fusion technique for neuroarthropathic feet: biomechanical analysis and rationale. Foot Ankle Int 1998;19(8):507–10.
57. Aiyer A, Russell NA, Pelletier MH, et al. The impact of nitinol staples on the compressive forces, contact area, and mechanical properties in comparison to a claw plate and crossed screws for the first tarsometatarsal arthrodesis. Foot Ankle Spec 2016;9(3):232–40.
58. Saxena A, Arthur WP, Ratnala D, et al. Arthrodesis in acute and chronic Lisfranc's patients: a retrospective cohort study. J Foot Ankle Surg 2021;22. S1067-2516(21)00351-3.
59. Jung HG, Myerson MS, Schon LC. Spectrum of operative treatments and clinical outcomes for atraumatic osteoarthritis of the tarsometatarsal joints. Foot Ankle Int 2007;28(4):482–9.
60. Rosemberg DL, Sposeto BR, Macedo RS, et al. Staged management of Lisfranc complex injury: case report and literature review. FussSprungg 2021;19(4): 218–28.
61. Halm JA, Rammelt S, Schepers T. Complex injuries of the foot and ankle: early and definite management. FussSprungg 2021;19(4):196–205.
62. Raikin SM, Schon LC. Arthrodesis of the fourth and fifth tarsometatarsal joints of the midfoot. Foot Ankle Int 2003;24(8):584–90.
63. Gougoulias N, Lampridis V. Midfoot arthrodesis. Foot Ankle Surg 2016;22(1): 17–25.

Medial Column Fusions in Flatfoot Deformities

Naviculocuneiform and Talonavicular

James A. Lendrum, MD, MPH, Kenneth J. Hunt, MD*

KEYWORDS

- Flatfoot deformity • Progressive collapsing flatfoot deformity
- Medial column arthrodesis • Naviculocuneiform arthrodesis
- Talonavicular arthrodesis • Deformity correction

KEY POINTS

- When treating flatfoot deformity, it is crucial to critically assess weight-bearing radiographs and address the deformity at the proper location.
- Naviculocuneiform arthrodesis is a reliable treatment for severe flatfoot deformity, demonstrating correction of flatfoot radiographic parameters and long-lasting results.
- Other components of flatfoot deformity can still be addressed when performing naviculocuneiform arthrodesis, such as soft tissue reconstruction and hindfoot alignment correction.
- Talonavicular arthrodesis also provides excellent correction of radiographic flatfoot parameters, however, at the expense of subtalar motion and with a nonunion rate estimated at 10% to 25%.
- Medial column arthrodesis can be especially useful in the revision setting, particularly when degenerative changes are present.

INTRODUCTION

Progressive collapsing foot deformity (PCFD) is a commonly encountered problem in foot and ankle surgery characterized by the hallmark features of hindfoot valgus, midfoot abduction, and forefoot varus.[1] Causes include degenerative, congenital, genetic, posttraumatic, as well as neuropathic and rheumatologic conditions. Common to all underlying causes is a loss of the longitudinal arch with attrition of the posterior tibialis tendon (PTT).[1–4] The spectrum of disease has been well described[5] and includes PTT inflammation, flexible flatfoot deformity, rigid deformity, and progressive deformity causing loss of ankle joint congruity and wear.

Department of Orthopedics, University of Colorado, 12631 East 17th Avenue, Mail Stop B202, Aurora, CO 80045, USA
* Corresponding author.
E-mail address: kenneth.j.hunt@cuanschutz.edu

Foot Ankle Clin N Am 27 (2022) 769–786
https://doi.org/10.1016/j.fcl.2022.08.006
1083-7515/22/© 2022 Elsevier Inc. All rights reserved.

The primary dynamic stabilizers of the medial column/longitudinal arch include the PTT, peroneus longus, and the windlass mechanism,[6] whereas the static stabilizers include first metatarsal length, spring ligament, plantar calcaneonavicular ligament, and deltoid ligament.[3] As a powerful inverter and plantarflexor, the PTT helps lock the transverse tarsal joints during gait.[7] Deficiency and attrition of the PTT lead to inability to lock the transverse tarsal joints, progressive strain on the medial soft stabilizers, and eventual collapse of the medial longitudinal arch with uncovering of the talus. This is worsened by the vector of pull of the Achilles tendon as the hindfoot falls into valgus, ultimately resulting in a rigid deformity in chronic cases. In order to accommodate the hindfoot valgus and maintain a plantigrade foot, the forefoot adapts with a varus deformity characterized by elevation of the first ray.[8] Patients often present with medial hindfoot pain in the region of the inflamed tendon; however, as deformity progresses, pain can present laterally as the calcaneus abuts the fibula.[2]

Some of the earliest procedures used to treat flatfoot deformity involved medial column fusions. The Miller procedure was first described for treatment of adolescent flatfoot in 1927, which involves naviculocuneiform (NC) and first tarsometatarsal (first TMT) arthrodesis with an osteoperiosteal flap for advancement of the medial static and dynamic stabilizers.[9] This was modified by Hoke[10–12] in 1931 and again by Caldwell in 1953, termed the "Durham-plasty." These original procedures required extensive soft tissue work and casting given the technological limitations of the time; however, with modern osseous fixation modalities, there is a need to revisit the modern role these procedures play in treatment of flatfoot deformity.[12,13]

CLINICAL EVALUATION OF PROGRESSIVE COLLAPSING FOOT DEFORMITY

Given the wide spectrum of stages and causes for PCFD, treatment can be quite complex and can vary substantially from patient to patient. In order to understand the available treatment options, providers must have keen knowledge of the clinical and radiographic presentation of flatfoot deformity. Patients typically have some degree of hindfoot valgus as well as forefoot abduction, which can be seen clinically as "too many toes" on the lateral foot when viewing the heel from behind. In addition, it is important to determine the ability of both the hindfoot and the forefoot deformities to correct passively. Patients often demonstrate difficulty with single-leg heel rise, PTT weakness, and gastrocnemius tightness with a Silfverskiöld test.[2,14]

Radiographically, it is important to obtain weight-bearing series of both the foot and the ankle for all patients with flatfoot deformity. These will typically demonstrate talonavicular (TN) undercoverage, break in talo–first-metatarsal angle (Meary angle) on both the anteroposterior (AP) and the lateral foot radiograph, loss of calcaneal pitch, and elevation of the first ray on lateral view. Severe deformities may even show valgus talar tilt at the ankle as the deltoid ligament fails.[2] Hindfoot alignment radiographs have been shown to be an accurate and measurable assessment of hindfoot valgus.[14] Weight-bearing computed tomographic (CT) scan is also becoming a helpful modality not only for detailing joint surfaces but also for demonstrating joint axes, particularly the subtalar (ST) joint.[14,15] Although MRI and ultrasound can play a role in determining the integrity of soft tissue structures such as the PTT or spring ligament, they have a limited role in the workup of moderate to severe disease.[2]

Originally described in 3 stages by Johnson and Strom[4] in 1989, the classification of flatfoot deformity has undergone several modifications,[5,16] with the Myerson modification being the most widely accepted. Stage I is PTT tendonitis presenting with medial pain but without deformity or functional limitation. Stage II is a flexible deformity with inability to perform a single-leg heel rise. This is further subdivided into IIA with less than 30% TN uncoverage and IIB with greater than 30% uncoverage. Bluman and colleagues[16] added a IIC subgroup, which consists of medial column instability. Stage III is a rigid deformity with severe pain and inability to perform a single-leg heel rise. Stage IV is the same as stage III with the addition of talar tilt in the ankle joint, again with A and B subdivisions based on rigidity/arthritis.[3,5,16] More recently, the term progressive collapsing foot deformity has been defined as a more descriptive classification system.[17]

GENERAL TREATMENT PRINCIPLES

Treatment of flatfoot deformity can be guided by the classification in that rigid or severe deformities require arthrodesis, and more flexible deformities can be treated via flexible correction with a combination of bony procedures and soft tissue reconstruction.[2] Nonoperative management can be quite successful for stage I or mild stage II deformity and includes a combination of tendon rest with anti-inflammatories, offloading orthotics, and physical therapy for strengthening and stretching.[18] However, when deciding between operative management options for flexible or rigid flatfoot deformity, an operative plan should be individually tailored to a patient's deformity components. Cotton[19] originally described the "triangle of support" created by the first and fifth metatarsal heads, and the plantar heel. The ultimate goal of any flatfoot correction is to create a painless, plantigrade foot.

Traditionally, hindfoot valgus can be treated with either a medial displacing calcaneal osteotomy (MDCO) or an ST fusion. Midfoot abduction can be managed with a combination of either lateral column lengthening (LCL) or calcaneocuboid (CC) distraction arthrodesis and medial soft tissue procedures such as PTT advancement, flexor digitorum longus (FDL) transfer, and spring ligament repair/reconstruction. Finally, first ray elevation/forefoot varus can be managed with medial cuneiform plantarflexion osteotomy (Cotton) or a plantarflexing first TMT arthrodesis.[1,2,7] Nearly all patients with flatfoot deformity can benefit from some form of Achilles tendon or gastrocnemius lengthening.[14] Flexibility of deformity, presence of arthritis, severity of deformity, and patients factors such as age/occupation all play a role in determining a treatment plan. One general principle of flatfoot treatment is that soft tissue procedures alone will ultimately fail if the underlying bony deformity is not simultaneously corrected.[1]

When assessing radiographs, it is vital to determine where the primary deformity is taking place, particularly on the lateral view. The break in the longitudinal arch, although classically described as taking place at the TN joint, can also occur at either the NC joint or the TMT joint. Instability of these joints can be identified with the presence of plantar gapping, which can be seen in **Fig. 1**A at the NC joint.[13,20,21] Failure to recognize joint sag and correction of the deformity at the proper location can lead to deformity recurrence and poor outcomes.[21,22] In addition, it is important to assess the magnitude of deformity, as significant deformities in the sagittal plane may not be correctable through joint-preserving surgeries such as a Cotton.[1] Although they play an important role in the treatment of flatfoot, first TMT fusion and Cotton osteotomy are not the focus of this article and will not be discussed further in detail.

The role of medial column arthrodesis in the treatment of PCFD is not entirely defined. The medial column arthrodesis is rarely an isolated procedure but is rather combined in most cases with other bone and soft tissue procedures. The goal of this review is to outline the role of medial column arthrodesis in PCFD, particularly TN and NC arthrodesis. The authors discuss the surgical considerations and postoperative management and review the outcomes as reported by available literature, in the context of complex case examples.

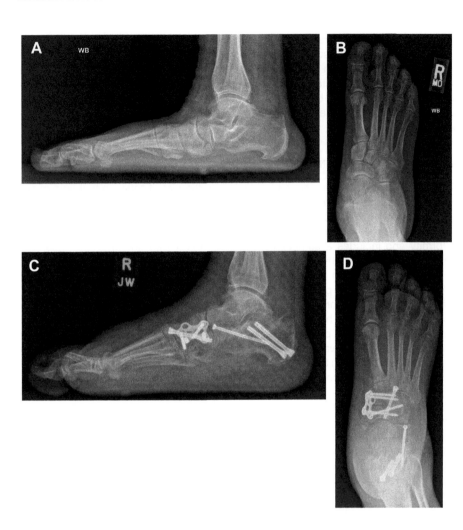

Fig. 1. (*A, B*) Preoperative AP and lateral weight-bearing foot radiographs showing PCFD with a primary sag at the NC joint with plantar gapping. (*C, D*) Postoperative AP and lateral weight-bearing foot radiographs following MDCO, LCL, and NC arthrodesis.

PREOPERATIVE/PREPROCEDURE PLANNING

As with any surgery, but particularly for flatfoot correction, it is important to tailor a surgical plan for each patient's deformity.[21] The traditional algorithms for flatfoot corrective surgeries have significant shortcomings.

Although a powerful corrective tool, LCL, typically indicated for correction of midfoot abduction, has been shown to have lower outcome scores when overcorrected. In addition, Thordarson and colleagues showed that length measurements of the lateral column are no different in patients with flat feet compared with patients without.[7,22,23] There is also debate as to the long-term consequences of increased pressures at the CC joint as a result of LCL.[7] The authors do not fully understand the long-term consequences of iatrogenically lengthening the lateral column. Regarding the medial column, traditional procedures, such as the Cotton or first

TMT arthrodesis, fail to address instability or degenerative changes at the NC and TN joints of the medial column.[21]

Another potential shortcoming involves the triple arthrodesis. Classically, patients with either severe flatfoot deformity or rigid deformity have been indicated for a triple arthrodesis, namely fusion of the ST, TN, and CC joints.[8] Although generally a successful procedure, it creates very rigid hindfoot and transverse tarsal joints, and unfortunately, deformity can still recur at joints distal to the fusion.[2] For example, if a patient has a severe flatfoot deformity, however, radiographs show significant sag at the NC joint (see **Fig. 1A**), and a triple arthrodesis may not be the best treatment option, as it does not fully address their deformity. In addition, combining a triple arthrodesis with a medial column procedure creates a very stiff foot that places significant stress on the ankle joint.[1,21,22]

A general principle for flatfoot surgery is attempting to achieve a painless, plantigrade foot while fusing the least number of joints possible.[8,12,24] Several studies have shown that NC arthrodesis consistently improves radiographic hindfoot alignment parameters, indicating there is a relationship between midfoot stability and hindfoot alignment.[13,22,25] The authors do not fully understand this relationship to date, but can potentially use this relationship to their advantage in sparing joints during flatfoot correction.

The authors' primary indications for including medial column arthrodesis in the treatment of flatfoot are the following:

- Moderate to severe deformity with instability of the NC joint[12,21]
- Severe, rigid deformity in the sagittal plane unlikely to correct with a Cotton or first TMT arthrodesis[1,22,26]
- Revision flatfoot correction with arthritic changes of the TN or NC joint
- NC arthrodesis in combination with flexible flatfoot correction (MDCO, LCL, FDL transfer, spring ligament repair/reconstruction)[22]

Caution should be taken when choosing to do medial column arthrodesis, especially in isolation, in the following situations: hypermobility/degenerative changes at adjacent joints, ankle joint instability or arthrosis, neuropathic and rheumatoid patients with significant bony loss, severe vascular disease, and smokers.[12,27] It is critical to only offer medial column arthrodesis to the properly indicated patient.

The authors discuss this further in a later section; however, it should be noted that hindfoot motion is intricately tied to TN motion. As a pseudo–ball-and-socket joint, the TN joint works in concert with the ST and CC joints to achieve triplanar motion. ST motion is particularly tied to TN motion. Biomechanical studies have shown that up to 80% to 98% of hindfoot motion and 75% of PTT excursion are lost with TN arthrodesis.[3,8,25,28] Therefore, it is rare in the authors' practice to perform an isolated TN arthrodesis without using an ST arthrodesis to aid in stability of the fusion and correct hindfoot alignment.

PROCEDURAL DETAILS AND TECHNIQUE
Positioning/Setup

Positioning is a critical portion of the case and is similar to any flatfoot correction. Patients are placed supine with a bump under the hip to rotate the knee and ankle to neutral. The authors typically use an elevation wedge or blanket stack under the knee and lower leg to help obtain lateral fluoroscopic views. It is important to have the patient distal enough on the table in order to have the foot and ankle free floating to be able to test simulated weight-bearing. A thigh tourniquet is placed and inflated to 250 mm Hg. Order of operations typically proceeds in a proximal to distal fashion given the downstream effect of deformity correction.

Procedural Technique

Equinus and hindfoot valgus

Nearly all patients with a flatfoot deformity will receive some form of Achilles or gastrocnemius lengthening. Patients with a positive Silfverskiöld test will receive a gastrocnemius recession, whereas those that are negative will receive a triple-cut tendo-Achilles lengthening.

In addition, patients with significant hindfoot valgus based on hindfoot alignment view will receive either an MDCO or an ST fusion. The authors perform their MDCO via minimally invasive (MIS) means using a small laterally based incision using an MIS bur. The authors use fluoroscopy and tactile feedback to confirm full release of the osteotomy site, aiming for 5 to 10 mm of displacement. The osteotomy is held with two 5.5-mm partially threaded cannulated screws placed through the heel. Details of the ST fusion are beyond the scope of this review; however, incision choice must be made carefully based on expected incisions for other planned work. The MIS nature of the authors' correction can be particularly helpful in terms of incision management. For ST fusion, the joint debridement can be performed arthroscopically if needed to help incision management. Once hindfoot alignment and equinus have been addressed, the authors then are able to proceed with medial column arthrodesis.

Talonavicular arthrodesis

The authors plan out a longitudinal medial-based incision. If needing to perform work on the PTT, the extensile nature of this approach extents from just distal to the tip of the medial malleolus to the medial aspect of the first TMT joint. Fluoroscopy should be used to mark out the portion of the incision that is desired for joint preparation/access. This approach should access the joints just dorsal to the PTT and plantar to the tibialis anterior (TA) tendon.

Once down to joint, the authors typically use a pin distractor or lamina spreader to help open up the TN joint. A combination of curette, rongeur, and osteotomes can be used to denude the cartilaginous surface. It is important to spend time removing the most plantar cartilage, as this will help correct the deformity in addition to improve fusion rates. The authors typically will use a small Kirschner wire to drill small holes throughout the newly denuded joint surface to help increase fusion surface area and stimulate bony growth. Once the bony surfaces have been prepared, bone graft can be inserted, and then the authors proceed with reduction of deformity, one of the most critical portions of the case. With the dorsolateral peritalar subluxation, it is important not only to rotate the navicular around the talus with lateral pressure on the talar head but also to correct the sagittal plane deformity with a dorsally directed force on the talus and a plantar-medial–directed force for the remaining foot.[3] Severe deformity may not be able to be corrected manually, and reduction clamps or pin distractors, such as the Hintermann, are powerful tools.[22] Once one is content with the reduction, this can be held in place with several large Kirschner wires, and reduction can be checked fluoroscopically using a footplate to help simulate weight-bearing and whether recreation of a plantigrade foot has been achieved. Fixation constructs can vary from cannulated screws alone, in combination with nitinol staples or plate/screw constructs.[8] Several examples are shown in the next section.

If desired, this approach facilitates work on medial soft tissue structures.[22] The authors prefer to use an absorbable suture, such as 0-Vicryl, to repair the spring ligament and will trim any diseased PTT. Given the PTT primarily works through TN motion, the authors do not routinely perform any tendon transfers during TN fusion, as they would have limited excursion with a successful fusion of this joint. Given the limited hindfoot motion associated with a TN arthrodesis, the authors will typically perform this in conjunction with an ST arthrodesis through either a sinus tarsi approach or an extension of the medially based incision depending on degree of deformity correction desired.

Naviculocuneiform arthrodesis

Although this joint can be accessed through a medial incision,[3] it is difficult to reach the more lateral portions of the NC joint. The authors therefore prefer to use a dorso-medial incision between the TA and extensor hallucis longus (EHL) tendons, having marked out the NC joint fluoroscopically. Care should be taken when dissecting in this region to avoid the neurovascular bundle, as aberrant anatomy can exist. Once down to NC joint, the cartilaginous surfaces can be prepared in a similar fashion to the TN joint. The authors prefer to denude all of the NC joints and intercuneiform joints, as this provides a more stable bony block for fusion, and the effect on motion is small, although leaving the lateral cuneiform unfused is perfectly acceptable.[3]

It is again important to remove the plantar cartilage and even a small portion of the bony surface, as this helps with deformity correction. Once the cartilage is removed, reduction of the NC joint proceeds in a similar fashion to the TN joint, taking care to assess the multiplanar correction fluoroscopically. This is typically accomplished via plantarflexion and adduction of the first ray to place in line with the navicular.[25] If needed, an osteotomy can be performed through the plantar portions of the joint to aid in deformity correction. Large K-wires can again be used for provisional fixation. Definitive fixation can consist of cannulated lag screws, nitinol staples, or a combination of these and a medially based plate/screw construct.[25]

Bone graft and fusion additives

Bone grafts and additives are a crucial portion of the case, from a biological perspective related to fusion, but also can be used to aid structurally. The authors commonly use autograft, harvesting from the calcaneus, proximal tibia, or iliac crest. If a structural autograft is necessary, the authors typically would choose iliac crest. However, it is more common in the authors' practice to use structural allograft in the setting of bone loss or severe deformity and supplement with local autograft/aspirate, demineralized bone matrix (DBM), or platelet-derived growth factor (PDGF).

Postoperative Management

Although maintaining motion for the nonfused joints is important, obtaining a solid bony fusion can be a challenge and should take priority.[12] Every immobilization period should be individualized; however, for the authors' medial column fusions, they typically recommend 8 to 12 weeks of non-weight-bearing and 2 to 6 weeks of strict immobilization.[7] Patients are splinted for the first 2 weeks for wound protection, and depending on the deformity severity, construct strength, and wound appearance can either continue in a splint or transition to a postoperative boot. Progressive weight-bearing typically starts in the boot with increasing 25% body weight weekly with help of the physical therapy team until full painless weight-bearing is achieved in a walking boot. Patients can transition out of the walking boot once painless full weight-bearing and solid bony fusion have been achieved without change in alignment or hardware integrity, typically between 3 and 4 months postoperatively.

MANAGEMENT/CASE DISCUSSION

Case 1: Flexible Flatfoot Correction with Naviculocuneiform Arthrodesis

Fig. 1A and B show the preoperative AP and lateral foot radiographs of a 61-year-old woman with semi-flexible flatfoot with severe deformity. Close scrutinization of the lateral radiograph demonstrates plantar gapping at the NC joint. This patient underwent flatfoot correction with gastrocnemius recession, MDCO with 2 × 5.5-mm partially threaded headless screws, LCL with an Evans bone block wedge, NC arthrodesis using a medially based plate/screw construct with additional middle cuneiform-navicular lag screw, PTT debridement, and spring ligament repair. All 3 cuneiform joints were prepared, and final healed radiographs can be seen in **Fig. 1**C and D, noting excellent correction of deformity with restoration of Meary angle, and coverage of the TN joint.

Case 2: Revision Flatfoot Correction with Medial Column Arthrodesis

The preoperative AP and lateral foot radiographs of a 66-year-old woman with flatfoot deformity following previous midfoot arthrodesis can be seen in **Fig. 2**A and B. In addition to the deformity through the NC joint, note the nonunion of the intercuneiform joint. She underwent flatfoot correction with gastrocnemius recession and NC arthrodesis using a medially based plate/screw construct spanning to the first metatarsal given the prior fusion. Second and third TMT joints were also included in the fusion mass as were all cuneiforms. Cancellous chips and DBM were used to supplement the fusion, as pannus was a concern regarding iliac crest bone grafting (ICBG) harvesting. Final healed radiographs can be seen in **Fig. 2**C and D, again noting solid correction of deformity with restoration of Meary angle, and improvement in calcaneal pitch.

Case 3: Revision Flatfoot Correction with Medial Column Arthrodesis Using Hybrid Fixation

Fig. 3A and B show the preoperative AP and lateral foot radiographs of a 34-year-old woman with mild flatfoot deformity following midfoot arthrodesis and a painful arthritic NC joint. She underwent flatfoot correction with gastrocnemius recession and NC arthrodesis using 3 retrograde screws across the fusion mass, an intercuneiform screw, and 2 additional nitinol staples across the NC joint. Cancellous chips mixed with DBM and PDGF were used to supplement the fusion. Final healed radiographs can be seen in **Fig. 3**C–E with solid fusion and correction of deformity.

Case 4: Double Arthrodesis for Flatfoot with Talonavicular Arthritic Changes

The preoperative AP and lateral foot radiographs of a 74-year-old woman with mild flatfoot deformity in the setting of significant talar subluxation and degenerative changes at the TN and ST joints can be seen in **Fig. 4**A and B. She underwent double arthrodesis involving the TN and ST joints. Two 5.5-mm partially threaded screws were used for the ST joint, whereas a combination of two 4.5-mm fully threaded screws and a medially based nitinol staple was used for the TN joint. Healed radiographs at 4 months postoperatively can be seen in **Fig. 4**C and D with solid fusion and correction of deformity. (Case and radiographic images courtesy of Steven L Haddad MD.)

Case 5: Talonavicular Arthrodesis Using a Medial Plate-Screw Construct

Fig. 5A and B show a different construct involving a medially based plate/screw construct for a TN arthrodesis in combination with an MDCO for flatfoot deformity and hindfoot valgus.

Case 6: Severe Flatfoot Deformity with Recurrence Following Double Arthrodesis

Fig. 6A and B depict the preoperative AP and lateral foot radiographs of an 86-year-old man with severe flatfoot deformity demonstrated by significant TN undercoverage, midfoot abduction, and significant declination of Meary angle. Given the severity of deformity, he underwent double arthrodesis involving the TN and ST joints. Three

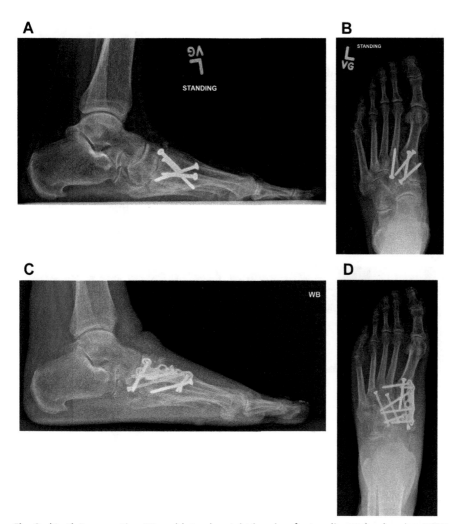

Fig. 2. (*A, B*) Preoperative AP and lateral weight-bearing foot radiographs showing PCFD following attempted midfoot arthrodesis and associated midfoot nonunion. (*C, D*) Eighteen-month postoperative AP and lateral weight-bearing foot radiographs following medial column fusion.

5.5-mm fully threaded screws were used for the ST joint, whereas again a combination of three 4.5-mm fully threaded screws and a medially based nitinol staple was used for the TN joint. Fluoroscopic views can be seen in **Fig. 6**C–E, demonstrating significant improvement in TN coverage, Meary angle, and midfoot abduction. Unfortunately, this patient's deformity recurred through the NC joint as shown at 6-month postoperative radiographs in **Fig. 6**F and G with healed TN and ST fusions. The patient was asymptomatic, and no further surgeries are planned.

Case 7: Traumatic Flatfoot Deformity with Talonavicular Nonunion and Deformity Recurrence

Fig. 7A and B show the preoperative AP and lateral foot radiographs of a 63-year-old man with severe posttraumatic flatfoot deformity with chronic dislocation of the TN

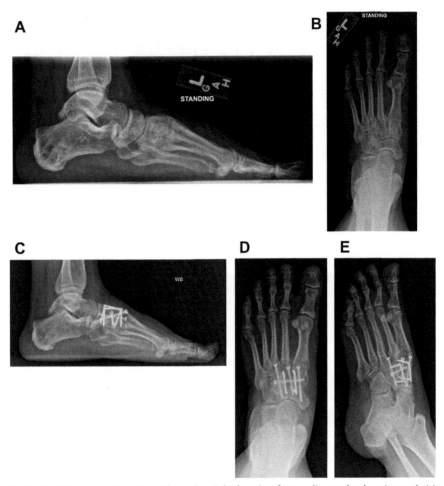

Fig. 3. (*A*, *B*) Preoperative AP and lateral weight-bearing foot radiographs showing arthritic change at the NC joint following successful midfoot fusion. (*C*, *D*, *E*) Eighteen-month post-operative AP, oblique, and lateral weight-bearing foot radiographs following medial column fusion.

joint, midfoot abduction, and significant loss of calcaneal pitch. Given the severity of deformity, he also underwent double arthrodesis involving the TN and ST joints. Two 7.0-mm fully partially screws were used for the ST joint, whereas three 4.5-mm partially threaded screws were used for the TN joint. Fluoroscopic views can be seen in **Fig. 7**C and D, demonstrating significant improvement in TN coverage, Meary angle, and midfoot abduction. ICBG and DBM were used to supplement the fusion. Unfortunately, this patient's deformity recurred via a nonunion of the TN joint as demonstrated by the broken hardware and lack of osseous bridging on weight-bearing CT and was additionally found to have arthritic changes to the tibiotalar joint as seen in **Fig. 7**E–G. This patient is planned to undergo revision deformity correction with revision TN arthrodesis with bone grafting, removal of ST hardware, and a total ankle replacement.

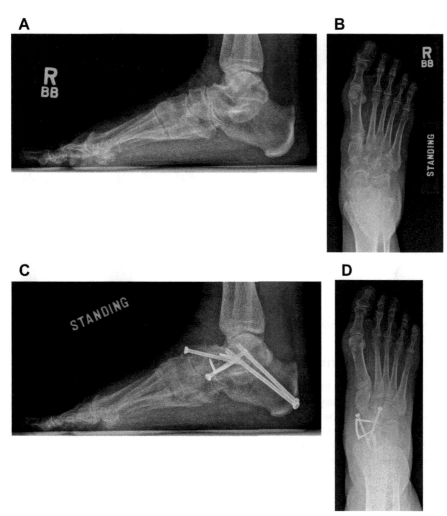

Fig. 4. (*A, B*) Preoperative AP and lateral weight-bearing foot radiographs showing PCFD with maintenance of arch height despite significant midfoot abduction and TN undercoverage. (*C, D*) Postoperative AP and lateral weight-bearing foot radiographs following double arthrodesis.

Case 8: Medial Column Arthrodesis in the Management of Charcot Reconstruction

Other indications for medial column arthrodesis include Charcot reconstruction. **Fig. 8**A–C demonstrate the initial preoperative AP and lateral juxtaposed with another preoperative lateral foot radiograph 6 months later (immediately preoperatively) of a 64-year-old man with Charcot arthropathy. Note the progressive collapse through the midfoot on **Fig. 8**C. This patient underwent Charcot reconstruction with midfoot biplanar osteotomy (plantarly and laterally) with TN, CC, and midfoot fusion with 7.2-mm medial column beam, MIS LDCO, claw toe correction, and open z-lengthening of Achilles. ICBG and cancellous chips were used. The patient healed well after 12-weeks strict non-weight-bearing and a progressive weight-bearing protocol thereafter. Final healed radiographs can be seen in **Fig. 8**D and E.

A   B

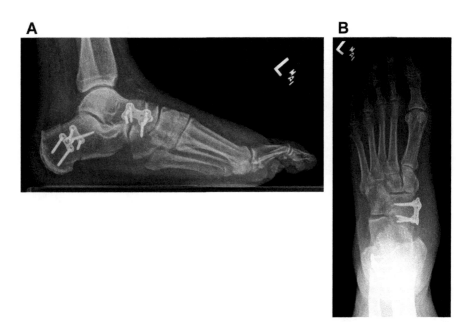

Fig. 5. (A, B) Postoperative weight-bearing foot radiographs following MDCO and TN arthrodesis for PCFD.

OUTCOMES IN LITERATURE

Available outcomes in the literature regarding medial column arthrodesis for correction of flatfoot are largely limited to several retrospective case series; however, they do highlight some of the complications alluded to in the case section.

In 2014, Ajis and Geary[28] presented a series of 33 feet that underwent isolated NC arthrodesis and reported significant improvement in pain scores and radiographic parameters, such as Meary angle and TN coverage. Although union occurred in 97% of patients, the average time to union was nearly 5 months.[29] Another study showed that the incidence of NC nonunion was approximately 7%; however, this increased as high as 15% when including additional joints such as the TMT.[30] A 15% nonunion risk may be unacceptably high in certain patient populations. Chan and colleagues[6] report the nonunion risk of NC arthrodesis as high as 12.5%.

Greisberg and colleagues[13] presented a series of 19 patients that had undergone isolated medial column arthrodesis (3 NC, 3 TMT, 13 combined NC/TMT) for flatfoot correction. They found 3 patients (15.7%) with nonunion (2 NC, 1 TMT). They also found significant improvements in hindfoot radiographic parameters with medial column arthrodesis. Meary angle improved from −19° to −3°; calcaneal pitch improved from 15° to 20°, and TN uncoverage improved from 28° to 14°. This indicates that isolated medial column fusion is a powerful corrective tool that has a profound effect on overall flatfoot parameters yet spares the hindfoot joints.

Barg and colleagues[12] present a series of 10 patients that underwent combined NC and ST arthrodesis. They found correction of all radiographic parameters, including TN subluxation, and they obtained successful arthrodesis radiographically between 8 and 12 weeks. Overall, patients had a high level of satisfaction with improved proprioception during walking/standing at 1 year. They only had 1 deformity recurrence, which they reported was likely secondary to incomplete correction of heel valgus, as it failed at the ST joint. There were no failures at the NC joint. Long-term follow-up of 22

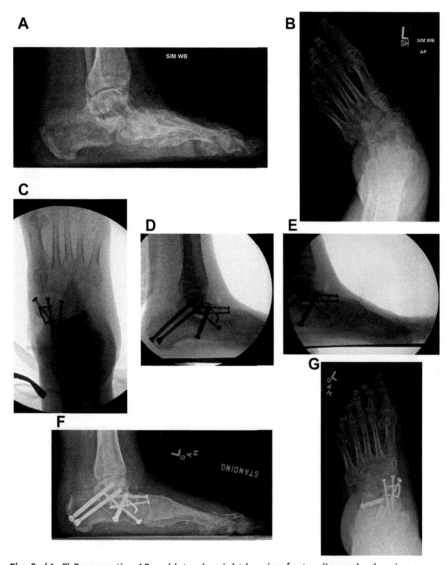

Fig. 6. (*A, B*) Preoperative AP and lateral weight-bearing foot radiographs showing severe PCFD with near dislocation of the TN joint. (*C, D, E*) Intraoperative AP and simulated weight-bearing laterals demonstrating excellent correction of the deformity. (*F, G*) Six-month postoperative AP and lateral weight-bearing foot radiographs following double arthrodesis with healed fusion sites and recurrence of deformity through the NC joint.

adolescent patients that had undergone the Miller procedure (average 12-year follow-up) reported 84% satisfaction with the dissatisfied group of 16% reporting continued symptoms. They did report a 21% nonunion rate, noting that most were asymptomatic.[31]

Camasta and colleagues[31] present a series of 51 flexible flatfoot patients that underwent isolated TN arthrodesis. Although they ultimately found 100% fusion rate, they reported 6 patients with adjacent joint breakdown (4 NC and 2 ST). Of patients, 88% were satisfied, with the 12% unsatisfied being the group with adjacent joint

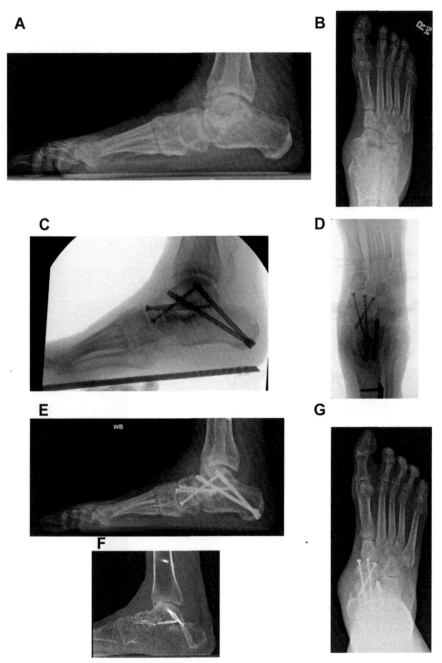

Fig. 7. (*A, B*) Preoperative AP and lateral weight-bearing foot radiographs showing post-traumatic flatfoot deformity and TN dislocation. (*C, D*) Intraoperative fluoroscopic AP and simulated weight-bearing laterals demonstrating excellent correction of the deformity. (*E–G*) Postoperative AP and lateral weight-bearing foot radiographs as well as a select cut from the sagittal weight-bearing CT demonstrate nonunion of the TN joint and arthritic changes to the tibiotalar joint following double arthrodesis.

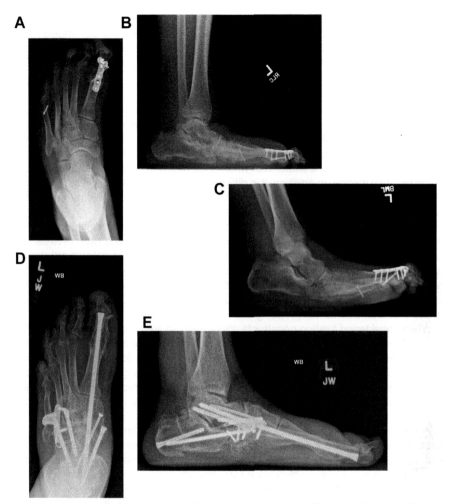

Fig. 8. (A, B) Preoperative AP and lateral weight-bearing foot radiographs showing Charcot arthropathy in setting of prior first MTP arthrodesis. (C) Repeat preoperative lateral foot radiograph; note the progressive collapse of the midfoot primarily through the NC joint. (D, E) Eighteen-month postoperative AP and lateral weight-bearing foot radiographs following Charcot reconstruction using medial column beaming.

breakdown and deformity recurrence.[32] Although the nonunion risk of NC arthrodesis is reported between 3% and 15%, the risk of nonunion associated with TN arthrodesis has been reported slightly higher between 10% and 25%.[3]

Harper and Tisdel[32] reviewed a series of 27 patients who underwent TN arthrodesis for treatment of flatfoot deformity and found 89% with no pain or pain only with heavy use. Only 2 patients had major reservations. All patients ultimately had a successful arthrodesis during the follow-up period of 12 to 27 months; however, there was 1 nonunion that required 2 additional grafting procedures. In addition, there were 5 patients with progression of adjacent joint arthrosis in their short follow-up period.[33] They concluded that TN arthrodesis provides excellent pain improvement and lasting stability.

Despite largely favorable results for NC arthrodesis, this is not the case for TN arthrodesis. Below and McCluskey[33] reported some less-favorable outcomes for isolated TN arthrodesis patients. Among 21 patients that underwent isolated TN fusion for symptomatic flatfoot, during their follow-up period, 8 (38.0%) developed radiographic ST arthrosis, 12 (57.1%) had ST pain, and most patients continued to have daily pain. There were 6 TN nonunions in this study (28.5%).[34]

SUMMARY

Based on the literature and the authors experience, with the appropriately selected patient, there is a role for medial column arthrodesis in the surgical management of flatfoot deformity. Although a triple arthrodesis is always a salvage option, medial column arthrodesis can be a useful tool when used appropriately and potentially spare some hindfoot motion. In addition, it is difficult to correct the first ray elevation through a triple arthrodesis, and significant deformity through the NC or TMT joint may be better suited with a medial column procedure.[12]

One of the biggest complications associated with these surgeries is nonunion. As with any fracture fixation or arthrodesis procedure, it is always a race between the bone healing or the fixation fatiguing. When considering medial column arthrodesis as a treatment option, maximizing both the biology and the fixation is paramount to a successful outcome. Although the exact makeup of fusion additives continues to be a topic of debate, the authors prefer autograft whenever possible. Structural allografts when mixed with the proper growth factors can also be useful.

When considering fixation constructs, this also is an area that lends itself to further clarity. Anecdotally, however, the NC and TN joints seem to be areas of high deforming force especially in the setting of severe or long-standing/rigid deformity. Using adjunctive procedures such as soft tissue reconstruction, hindfoot alignment osteotomies or arthrodesis, and equinus release is advised to help prevent recurrence. Robust, rigid fixation is also advised whether it be a plate/screw construct, using nitinol staple adjuncts, or hybrid fixation models.

In the authors' experience, isolated TN arthrodesis has limited indications, as it severely hinders hindfoot motion and has a high nonunion risk. Although TN arthrodesis can successfully correct alignment parameters, patients have significant stiffness, and there is a high complication rate. Nevertheless, there is certainly a role for double arthrodesis (TN + ST) in the setting of severe/fixed deformity.[12,27]

NC arthrodesis may have broader applications, as it can be combined with hindfoot alignment/arthrodesis procedures and maintain motion at the TN joint while still correcting deformity.[21] NC arthrodesis is a viable option in the setting of instability at the NC joint, sagittal plane deformity unlikely to correct with Cotton/first TMT arthrodesis procedure, or in combination with other flatfoot modalities (MDCO, LCL, FDL transfer, spring ligament repair/reconstruction).[22]

CLINICS CARE POINTS

- When treating flatfoot deformity, it is crucial to critically assess weight-bearing radiographs and address the deformity at the proper location.
- Naviculocuneiform arthrodesis is a reliable treatment for severe flatfoot deformity, demonstrating correction of flatfoot radiographic parameters and long-lasting results.
- Other components of flatfoot deformity can still be addressed when performing naviculocuneiform arthrodesis, such as soft tissue reconstruction and hindfoot alignment correction.

- Talonavicular arthrodesis also provides excellent correction of radiographic flatfoot parameters, however, at the expense of subtalar motion and with a nonunion rate estimated at 10% to 25%.
- Medial column arthrodesis can be especially useful in the revision setting, particularly when degenerative changes are present.

DISCLOSURE

There are no disclosure to be stated for the purpose of this article. The authors above have no commercial or financial conflicts of interest. The authors have nothing to disclose.

REFERENCES

1. McCormick JJ, Johnson JE. Medial column procedures in the correction of adult acquired flatfoot deformity. Foot Ankle Clin 2012;17(2):283–98.
2. Abousayed MM, Alley MC, Shakked R, et al. Adult-acquired flatfoot deformity: etiology, diagnosis, and management. JBJS Rev 2017;5(8):e7.
3. Cohen BE, Ogden F. Medial column procedures in the acquired flatfoot deformity. Foot Ankle Clin 2007;12(2):287–99.
4. Johnson KA, Strom DE. Tibialis posterior tendon dysfunction. Clin Orthop Relat Res 1989;239:196–206.
5. Myerson MS. Adult acquired flatfoot deformity: treatment of dysfunction of the posterior tibial tendon. Instr Course Lect 1997;46:393–405.
6. Chan F, Bowlby MA, Christensen JC. Medial column biomechanics: nonsurgical and surgical implications. Clin podiatric Med Surg 2020;37(1):39–51.
7. Hunt KJ, Farmer RP. The Undercorrected Flatfoot Reconstruction. Foot Ankle Clin 2017;22(3):613–24.
8. Johnson JE, Yu JR. Arthrodesis techniques in the management of stage II and III acquired adult flatfoot deformity. Instructional course lectures 2006;55:531–42.
9. Miller OL. A plastic flat foot operation. J Bone Joint Surg Am 1927;9:84–91.
10. Hoke M. An operation for the correction of extremely relaxed flat feet. J Bone Joint Surg Am 1931;13:773–83.
11. Caldwell GD. Surgical correction of relaxed flatfoot by the Durham flatfoot plasty. Clin Orthop 1953;2:221–6.
12. Barg A, Brunner S, Zwicky L, et al. Subtalar and naviculocuneiform fusion for extended breakdown of the medial arch. Foot Ankle Clin 2011;16(1):69–81.
13. Greisberg J, Assal M, Hansen ST Jr, et al. Isolated medial column stabilization improves alignment in adult-acquired flatfoot. Clin Orthopaedics Relat Research® 2005;435:197–202.
14. Conti MS, Garfinkel JH, Ellis SJ. Outcomes of reconstruction of the flexible adult-acquired flatfoot deformity. Orthop Clin 2020;51(1):109–20.
15. Haleem AM, Pavlov H, Bogner E, et al. Comparison of deformity with respect to the talus in patients with posterior tibial tendon dysfunction and controls using multiplanar weight-bearing imaging or conventional radiography. J Bone Joint Surg Am 2014;96(8):e63.
16. Bluman EM, Title CI, Myerson MS. Posterior tibial tendon rupture: a refined classification system. Foot Ankle Clin 2007;12(2):233–49.
17. Myerson MS, Thordarson DB, Johnson JE, et al. Classification and nomenclature: progressive collapsing foot deformity. Foot Ankle Int 2020;41(10):1271–6.

18. Alvarez RG, Marini A, Schmitt C, et al. Stage I and II posterior tibial tendon dysfunction treated by a structured nonoperative management protocol: an orthosis and exercise program. Foot Ankle Int 2006;27(1):2–8.

19. Cotton FJ. Foot statics and surgery. N Engl J Med 1936;353–62.

20. Kadakia AR, Kelikian AS, Barbosa M, et al. Did failure occur because of medial column instability that was not recognized, or did it develop after surgery? Foot Ankle Clin 2017;22(3):545–62.

21. Metzl JA. Naviculocuneiform Sag in the Acquired Flatfoot: What to Do. Foot Ankle Clin 2017;22(3):529–44.

22. Kang S, Charlton TP, Thordarson DB. Lateral column length in adult flatfoot deformity. Foot Ankle Int 2013;34(3):392–7.

23. Jack EA. Naviculo-cuneiform fusion in the treatment of flat foot. J Bone Joint Surg Br 1953;35-B(1):75–82.

24. Jordan TH, Rush SM, Hamilton GA, et al. Radiographic outcomes of adult acquired flatfoot corrected by medial column arthrodesis with or without a medializing calcaneal osteotomy. J foot Ankle Surg 2011;50(2):176–81.

25. Johnson JE. Plantarflexion opening wedge cuneiform-1 osteotomy for correction of fixed forefoot varus. Tech Foot Ankle Surg 2004;3:2–8.

26. Fortin PT. Posterior tibial tendon insufficiency: Isolated fusion of the talonavicular joint. Foot Ankle Clin 2001;6(1):137–51.

27. Astion DJ, Deland JT, Otis JC, et al. Motion of the hindfoot after simulated arthrodesis. JBJS 1997;79(2):241–6.

28. Ajis A, Geary N. Surgical technique, fusion rates, and planovalgus foot deformity correction with naviculocuneiform fusion. Foot Ankle Int 2014;35(3):232–7.

29. Ford LA, Hamilton GA. Naviculocuneiform arthrodesis. Clin Podiatr Med Surg 2004;21(1):141–56.

30. Fraser RK, Menelaus MB, Williams PF, et al. The Miller procedure for mobile flat feet. Journal of bone and joint surgery. British volume 1995;77(3):396–9.

31. Camasta CA, Menke CR, Hall PB. A review of 51 talonavicular joint arthrodesis for flexible pes valgus deformity. J Foot Ankle Surg 2010;49:113–8.

32. Harper MC, Tisdel CL. Talonavicular arthrodesis for the painful adult acquired flatfoot. Foot Ankle Int 1996;17(11):658–61.

33. Below S McCluskey. Isolated talonavicular arthrodesis for posterior tibial tendon dysfunction and degenerative joint disease of the talonavicular joint. In Read at the Annual Summer Meeting of the American Orthopaedic Foot and Ankle Society (pp. 12-14). July 12-14, 2002. Traverse City, MI.

34. Pedowitz WJ, Kovatis P. Flatfoot in the adult. J Am Acad Orthop Surg 1995;3(5):293–302.

Management of the Subtalar Joint Following Calcaneal Fracture Malunion

Benjamin J. Ebben, MD[a,b,*], Mark Myerson, MD[c]

KEYWORDS

- Calcaneus malunion • Subtalar arthrosis • Distraction arthrodesis
- In situ arthrodesis • Calcaneofibular abutment • Lateral wall exostectomy
- Calcaneus fracture • Calcaneus osteotomy

KEY POINTS

- Posttraumatic subtalar joint arthrosis is often a consequence of calcaneus fracture malunion.
- Calcaneus fracture malunions have consistent patterns of deformity, typically involving widening and shortening of the heel.
- Other secondary pain-generators frequently coexist with subtalar joint arthrosis and must be considered.
- Joint-preserving and joint-fusing surgical techniques are available.

BACKGROUND

Calcaneal fractures account for roughly 1% to 2% of all fractures but are the most fractured tarsal bone. About 75% of these are intra-articular, involving the subtalar joint. Men are affected more often than women. These injuries are associated with significant morbidity, functional disability, and negative socioeconomic impact. They are typically incurred because of high-energy trauma, such as a motor vehicle collision, or falls from height. They are often accompanied by substantial soft tissue injury, which heavily dictates the treatment algorithm along with fracture displacement and individual patient risk factors. Historically, there has been considerable controversy surrounding the treatment of these fractures with temporal trends advocating entirely noninvasive closed management and others favoring maximally invasive open

[a] Department of Orthopedic Surgery, University of Colorado School of Medicine, 12631 East 17th Avenue, Room 4508, Aurora, CO 80045, USA; [b] Bellin Health Titletown Sports Medicine and Orthopedics, 1970 South Ridge Road, Green Bay, WI 54304, USA; [c] University of Colorado, Foot and Ankle Clinics of N. America, Steps2Walk, 11026 East Crestline Circle, Englewood, CO 80111, USA
* Corresponding author.
E-mail address: benjaminebben@gmail.com

Foot Ankle Clin N Am 27 (2022) 787–803
https://doi.org/10.1016/j.fcl.2022.08.001
foot.theclinics.com

anatomic reduction and internal fixation through extensile surgical approaches. These vastly contrasting management strategies reflect 2 competing goals particularly relevant to calcaneal fracture treatment: minimization of secondary soft tissue trauma and reestablishment of normal calcaneal morphology. Although surgical calcaneus fracture treatment classically has a high rate of, sometimes, devastating wound complications, there is value in recreating the anatomy to maximize hindfoot biomechanics and function. As the knowledge regarding soft tissue handling techniques and percutaneous reduction and fixation techniques has evolved, the optimal treatment likely involves a hybrid approach, and the pendulum currently rests somewhere in the middle on the treatment spectrum.

Late sequelae after calcaneus fractures are common even despite appropriate initial management. Poorer patient outcomes are consistently associated with malunion and residual hindfoot deformity. Painful posttraumatic subtalar arthrosis may occur following intra-articular calcaneus fractures in the setting of seemingly minor persistent joint surface incongruity. It has been shown that only 2 mm of articular displacement involving the posterior facet of the subtalar joint leads to abnormal joint forces and inferior clinical outcomes.[1] Of note, earlier investigations have identified variables predictive of late subtalar arthrodesis surgery. Csizy and colleagues[2] reported a 6-fold increase in the need for late secondary subtalar arthrodesis in calcaneus fractures treated conservatively compared with operative fixation. The subtalar joint is central to normal hindfoot biomechanics, especially with inversion and eversion. This motion is critical for shock absorption during heel strike and adaptation of the hindfoot during midstance. Subtalar arthrosis restricts this coronal plane motion and may lead to altered gait mechanics and, in particular, difficulty with ambulation on uneven surfaces. Moreover, abduction and adduction through the transverse tarsal joint also depends on normal subtalar joint biomechanics. Mann and colleagues[3] reported a 50% reduction in transverse plane motion across the Chopart joint, relative to the contralateral side, in patients who underwent unilateral isolated subtalar arthrodesis.

Symptomatic articular malunion and posttraumatic subtalar arthrosis often occurs in association with a combination of additional pain sources related to classic calcaneus fracture malalignment patterns and the resulting pathomechanics. Owing to the divergence of the talar and calcaneal mechanical axes through the subtalar joint, high-energy axial loads typically produce a medial shear sagittal plane primary fracture line through the calcaneus generating a superomedial fracture fragment containing the sustentaculum tali and a posterolateral fragment containing the calcaneal tuberosity. The tuberosity fragment typically translates superiorly and laterally relative to the sustentaculum. Variable secondary and tertiary fracture lines often exist. Multiple calcaneus fracture classification schemes have been developed. The most widely used is that by Sanders and colleagues,[4] which is based on the number and location of fracture lines involving the posterior facet of the subtalar joint on coronal computed tomography (CT). The rapid deceleration fracture mechanism consistently leads to some degree of lateral calcaneal wall blowout as well. Malunions, therefore, often feature a widened hindfoot, which may lead to calcaneofibular abutment, sural neuritis and peroneal tendonitis, tearing or instability. Collapse of the posterior facet into the sparsely trabeculated neutral triangle portion of the calcaneus body commonly results in hindfoot shortening and flattening of the longitudinal arch, which is manifested radiographically by a decreased calcaneal height, decreased calcaneal pitch, and a more horizontal talar declination angle. These malunions produce abnormal tibiotalar joint biomechanics and can lead to loss of ankle dorsiflexion, anterior impingement, and, ultimately, tibiotalar arthrosis. In addition, descent of the malleoli, which is more accurately a relative shortening of the hindfoot, can lead to footwear irritation.

Beyond the osseous problems of hindfoot deformity and posttraumatic subtalar arthrosis, there are essential considerations involving the status of the soft tissue envelope, which weigh heavily on treatment strategy. **Fig. 1** depicts a scenario where the presence of superficial infection warranted the staged management of a calcaneus fracture malunion. On the lateral side of the ankle and hindfoot, for example, the peroneal tendons are frequently irritated and torn from lateral wall exostosis or frankly dislocated from rupture of the superior peroneal retinaculum at the time of the initial injury. In the setting of previous calcaneal fracture surgery, the surgical approach used and associated fibrosis and adhesions, as well as the presence of retained orthopedic hardware, will influence secondary surgical options. Sural neuritis or entrapment is not an uncommon sequalae and may necessitate concomitant treatment. Considerations on the medial side include tethering of the flexor hallucis longus and compression of the tibial nerve and its branches in the tarsal tunnel, which can be a tension-related phenomenon is the setting of severe deformity. In addition, posteriorly, the Achilles-gastrocnemius-soleus complex must be assessed for the presence of equinus contracture, which may occur in the presence of longstanding relative hindfoot shortening. There may also be sympathetic-mediated pain syndromes at play. Although the focus of this review is on the management of the subtalar joint following calcaneus fracture malunion, it is in rare scenarios that the subtalar arthrosis can be addressed in isolation. All of the previously stated potential symptom generators and secondary issues must be considered when structuring an individualized treatment approach for these patients.

PATIENT ASSESSMENT AND NONOPERATIVE MANAGEMENT

The evaluation of a patient with a painful hindfoot and history of calcaneus fracture begins with a physical examination. The general shape of the heel should be assessed for

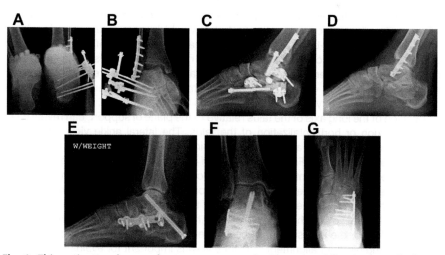

Fig. 1. This patient's calcaneus fracture was treated with external fixation initially (A–C). They presented with superficial skin infection 7 weeks following the procedure. In situ subtalar arthrodesis was staged. External fixator removal demonstrated the extent of the problem including the comminution involving the calcaneocuboid joint (D). Cancellous bone graft was used as a void filler in the body of the calcaneus as well as an augment in the calcaneocuboid joint. A long plate used to simultaneously fix the calcaneus and the calcaneocuboid arthrodesis. The plate also served to contain the cancellous graft (E–G).

widening and shortening compared with the contralateral side, if uninjured. Indirect findings associated with the loss of calcaneal height may include malleolar irritation indicative of relative descent and footwear conflict. In the setting of previous open reduction and internal fixation, surgical scar location and configuration should be noted. About 8.5% of calcaneus fractures are open,[5] typically medially, and the skin overlying the medial hindfoot should be assessed thoroughly as well. Asymmetric plantar callosities, particularly involving the lateral midfoot, suggest a varus hindfoot malunion. Examination of the sole of the shoe may also reveal abnormal or asymmetric wear patterns consistent with abnormal hindfoot biomechanics. Standing hindfoot alignment, when viewed from posteriorly, is critical in detection of deformity. The ankle, subtalar, and transverse tarsal joints are tested for range of motion, crepitus, stability, and pain. Ankle dorsiflexion can be mechanically limited by the collapse of the posterior facet and horizontalization of the talus. It may be difficult to differentiate this from an Achilles tendon or gastrocnemius contracture.

It is common for pain to be elicited with palpation over the sinus tarsi in the case of subtalar arthrosis or slightly posteriorly in the subfibular region in cases of calcaneo-fibular impingement. If possible, this should be differentiated from pain overlying the peroneal tendons or sural nerve. Resisted hindfoot eversion should be tested in addition to the stability of the peroneal tendons with circumduction of the hindfoot. On the medial side, flexion of the hallux should be confirmed to document excursion of the flexor hallucis longus tendon. A meticulous neurological examination may reveal dysesthesia or paresthesia in the sural nerve and/or posterior tibial nerve distributions. Electrophysiologic testing may be considered to further analyze these findings. Signs of poor perfusion or nonpalpable pulses should trigger additional vascular studies.

During nonoperative treatment and preoperative workup, diagnostic and potentially therapeutic corticosteroid or anesthetic injections can be used to confirm symptomatic contributors to patients' overall pain and dysfunction. For example, targeted injections into the subtalar joint can be used to differentiate lateral hindfoot pain secondary to peroneal tendinitis versus sinus tarsi impingement or calcaneofibular abutment.

Standard radiographic examination includes weight-bearing anteroposterior views of the ankle and weight-bearing anteroposterior and lateral views of the foot. A multitude of parameters are considered useful in the radiographic analysis of a calcaneus fracture malunion. Bohler's angle and the critical angle of Gissane are direct calcaneus morphologic measures of posterior facet height and displacement. The talus-first metatarsal angle (Meary's angle) and the talus declination angle, which measures the position of the long axis of the talus relative to the plane of support, can reveal relative dorsiflexion or horizontalization of the talus. The lateral ankle view may show osteophytes or asymmetric anterior tibiotalar joint space thinning when the talus declination angle is decreased (**Fig. 2**). Abutment of the lateral calcaneus in the subfibular region can be seen on the anteroposterior view of the ankle. Calcaneal pitch angle may be decreased and indicative of relative elevation of the tuberosity fragment. Talocalcaneal height is the distance from the dome of the talus to the base of the calcaneus and will be decreased in a shortened malunited hindfoot. An axial or Harris heel view is recommended for the assessment of heel widening and varus or valgus malunion. A weight-bearing hindfoot alignment or Cobey view is important for evaluating tibiocalcaneal alignment. Broden's views can supplement the radiographic evaluation and are useful for evaluating intra-articular step-offs involving the posterior facet.

Ultimately, calcaneus fracture malunions involve complex 3-dimensional deformities and advanced imaging is always necessary to guide treatment decisions. CT has become routine and should be protocolized for the hindfoot, specifically. Stephens and Sanders were the first to develop a calcaneal malunion classification

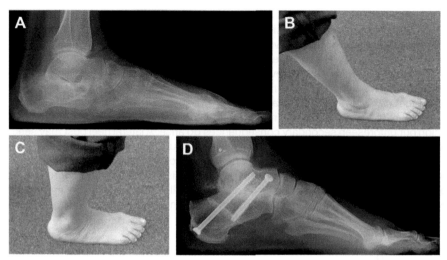

Fig. 2. Lateral standing radiograph of a patient with a calcaneus fracture malunion (*A*). This malunion features some posterior facet joint depression as well as a marked decrease in the talar declination angle. There are small anterior ankle osteophytes suggesting bony impingement. However, note the clinical images showing relatively well-preserved ankle range of motion with asymptomatic dorsiflexion past neutral (*B*, *C*). This patient underwent an in situ subtalar arthrodesis with a medial displacement calcaneal osteotomy. Note the radiographic correction of the pes planovalgus deformity and talar declination angle (*D*).

system and treatment algorithm based on CT after observing consistent deformity patterns in nonoperatively treated injuries.[6] In this system, type 1 malunions include lateral wall bulging and far lateral subtalar arthrosis without calcaneal deformity. These were treated with exostectomy and far lateral joint debridement. Type 2 malunions feature lateral exostosis and more significant central and lateral subtalar arthrosis with minimal (<10°) calcaneal deformity in the coronal plane. These were treated with exostectomy and in situ subtalar arthrodesis. Type 3s differ with addition of significant coronal plane deformity, and an extra-articular osteotomy was added to the exostectomy and subtalar fusion. Although useful, this classification scheme does not capture all malunion patterns including the fairly common problem of posterior facet collapse and loss of calcaneal height. Zwipp and Rammelt subsequently expanded on this classification system to address these shortcomings and recommended surgical solutions.[7]

The indications for weight-bearing CT have broadened dramatically since the arrival of this technology. There may be useful applications in the setting of calcaneus fracture malunion management. Welck and Myerson described the value of evaluating deformity and bony impingement patterns in a load-bearing position before treating a patient with a calcaneus malunion with a bone block subtalar distraction arthrodesis.[8]

MRI is not used routinely in the evaluation of a calcaneus fracture malunion but may be considered if there is suspicion for infection or avascular necrosis. MRI can provide a detailed assessment of articular cartilage thickness and may also be applied when determining the appropriateness of various subtalar joint preservation surgeries. Finally, MRI is the diagnostic of choice for some of the soft tissue sequalae associated with calcaneus fractures such as peroneal tendon tears or dislocation.

Conservative treatment can be attempted for calcaneus fracture malunion. This may be accomplished through activity modification, footwear adjustments, orthotics and immobilization, or bracing. These are supportive measures aimed at limiting motion in diseased articulations and opposing underlying deformity through extrinsic means. In general, hindfoot eversion and inversion will be painful in an arthritic subtalar joint and patients will avoid walking on uneven surfaces or will prefer coronal plane support in these situations. This can be provided to some extent with a University of California Berkeley Lab foot orthosis but more proximal support may be needed with rigid ankle-foot orthoses and custom lace up Arizona braces. Custom orthotics with medial or lateral heel posting can play a role in counteracting a varus or valgus hindfoot malunion but unforeseen secondary consequences do arise. A lateral heel post may seem reasonable for a patient with a varus malunion but could exacerbate symptoms of calcaneofibular impingement; for example, periodic injections can be used for therapeutic purposes. There may be cases where surgery is contraindicated such as in a patient with peripheral vascular disease, uncontrolled diabetes, or an irreparably compromised soft tissue envelope. Supportive treatment will be the mainstay in these circumstances.

OPERATIVE MANAGEMENT
Joint Preservation

In situations of relatively well-preserved overall calcaneus morphology and painful subtalar arthritic disease, motion-preserving joint-sparing surgical approaches may be considered. Some of these techniques will not correct any underlying deformity or biomechanical aberrances and, therefore, are indicated only in select cases. Overall, the results with subtalar joint salvage procedures have been favorable, although with relatively short-term follow-up. A few studies, which are discussed below, have reported the use of arthroscopic debridement of the subtalar joint to treat late sequelae following intra-articular calcaneus fractures. Subtalar arthroscopy is minimally invasive and can typically be accomplished through 3 small lateral hindfoot portal incisions. There is minimal risk for wound complications even in the setting of previous open calcaneus fracture treatment and early postoperative motion is facilitated. The technique typically affords examination of the posterior facet. Retained hardware can be left in place unless symptomatic or intra-articular.

Arthroscopic treatments

Elgafy performed subtalar arthroscopic debridement in a consecutive series of 10 patients with persistent subfibular pain at an average of 14 months following open reduction and internal fixation of an intra-articular calcaneus fracture.[9] Only cases with mild posttraumatic degenerative changes were deemed appropriate for inclusion, as determined by preoperative plain radiographs and CT. The joint was confirmed as the source of pain by at least partial improvement after subtalar local anesthetic injection. The subtalar arthroscopy was combined with additional extra-articular procedures in most cases, including peroneal tenolysis, lateral wall exostectomy, and tarsal tunnel release. The authors found that at an average of almost 17 months of follow-up, 80% of patients had considerable pain relief requiring no further treatments or reoperation. Two patients had persistent pain and required subsequent subtalar arthrodesis during the study period. Of note, both patients had Outerbridge grade IV chondromalacia of the subtalar joint at the time of arthroscopic inspection. In a similarly designed investigation, Lee and colleagues[10] performed subtalar arthroscopic releases without any other concomitant procedures in a series of 17 patients at an average of 11.3 months following calcaneus fracture injury for the indication of pain secondary to stiffness. Radiologic criteria were strict and patients were offered arthroscopy only if posterior facet articular incongruity measured less than 2 mm, and there was no evidence of joint space narrowing on plain radiographs and CT. At a mean follow-up of 16.8 months, 14 patients (82%) reported being "very satisfied" or "satisfied" with their treatment and underwent no further local injections or surgical management during the study period. Pain persisted in 3 "dissatisfied" patients and 2 required subsequent subtalar arthrodesis. Interestingly, all dissatisfied patients had grade 3 or 4 cartilage damage at the time of arthroscopy based on the International Cartilage Repair Society classification system. Subtalar motion, measured by goniometer, improved in all patients and was rated as normal or only mildly restricted (75%–100% of the contralateral side) in most patients at final follow-up. Based on the findings of the above and other small retrospective studies, subtalar arthroscopy may be an effective treatment of posttraumatic arthrosis in instances of minimal articular incongruity and limited joint space narrowing. Results have been poor with a high rate of conversion to arthrodesis with higher grade cartilage degeneration at the time of arthroscopy. Nonetheless, it is difficult to isolate the effectiveness of arthroscopic debridement, by itself, because this has historically been combined with additional extra-articular procedures especially in the setting of calcaneus fracture malunion.

Interposition arthroplasty

Interpositional arthroplasty techniques have been described for the subtalar joint. To the best of our knowledge, there has been a single publication using this technique for the indication of calcaneus fracture malunion. Kim and colleagues[11] reported on their clinical results using autologous tensor fascia lata and posterior ankle fat interposition grafts to avoid arthrodesis in a group of 22 patients with posttraumatic subtalar joint arthritis following calcaneus fracture. The subtalar joint was approached through an Ollier or extensile lateral incision, and the authors described a percutaneous technique for securing the autograft medially. At 17 months, the authors noted significant improvements in American Orthopedic Foot and Ankle Society (AOFAS) hindfoot and Visual Analog Scale (VAS) scores, and 73% of subjects reported excellent subjective satisfaction ratings. However, this was a small case series with short-term follow-up and no commentary on the extent of preoperative subtalar arthrosis or malunion, so limited conclusions can be made. In general, the use of interpositional grafts for the treatment of arthritic load-bearing joints is still experimental.

Calcaneus osteotomy

When a calcaneal malunion features a large articular incongruency, and it is diagnosed at a stage where the articular cartilage is still normal thickness and presumed healthy, corrective calcaneal osteotomy through the malunited fracture site may be undertaken to salvage the joint and preserve subtalar motion and maximize limb function.[12] Preoperative assessment with CT is recommended in this case to characterize the course of the malunited fracture line, define articular displacement, and to plan the corrective osteotomy. MRI may also be indicated to confirm the status of the articular surfaces. If diffuse cartilage damage is detected intraoperatively or on preoperative MRI, despite relatively maintained joint space on plain radiographs and CT, then corrective osteotomy should be abandoned for arthrodesis. In the setting of previous calcaneus fracture open reduction and internal fixation, some or all retained hardware will need to be removed to facilitate malunited fragment mobilization and reduction.

Yu and colleagues[13] reported on their results using corrective, mostly tongue-type, osteotomies for 26 calcaneus fracture malunions treated 5.7 months after injury. Patients in this series had mild to no osteoarthritis with near normal cartilage appearance on plain radiographs, CT, and intraoperative visual inspection. Most of these patients had been treated conservatively for their initial injury, which explains the presence of large articular displacement. It is important to note that both the authors and patients were prepared for a conversion to arthrodesis if intraoperative cartilage findings were found to be discordant with preoperative imaging. The procedures were performed through an extensile lateral approach, and following the elevation of the posterior facet, the authors used bone blocks fashioned from the lateral wall exostectomy or tri-cortical iliac crest autograft as structural void filler. In cases where the thalamic portion of the calcaneus was elevated more than 1.5 cm after correction, the authors had difficulty closing the incision and used acute skin flap transfer and dermatoplasty in 2 cases. After 2 years of follow-up 85% of patients were satisfied and had returned to preinjury employment and activities. AOFAS hindfoot scores improved significantly. Radiographic calcaneus morphologic measures were recreated close to anatomic. A single patient had persistent pain, restricted motion, and progressive subtalar arthritis and was converted to a subtalar arthrodesis in the study period. No wound complications were reported. The experience of Yu and colleagues highlights the importance of surgical approach planning. When calcaneal height is reestablished through reconstructive osteotomy, transverse or horizontal limbs of hindfoot surgical exposures are subject to tension during and after closure and are at risk for wound complications. If possible, this should be avoided. This concept will be further elaborated on later in this review when discussing distraction subtalar arthrodesis.

Rammelt published on joint-sparing corrective osteotomies in a smaller series (n = 5) of patients but with longer follow-up out to 4.1 years. These patients had healed malunited intra-articular calcaneus fractures and underwent correction at a mean of 12 weeks after the original injury.[14] Subjective satisfaction was reported in each case and all patients denied limitations during activities of daily living and at work. AOFAS scores were significantly improved from 19 preoperatively to 81.2 at final follow-up. These functional improvements occurred despite the progression to radiographic posttraumatic subtalar arthritis in 3 out of 5 patients. Of note, 2 patients underwent reoperations involving implant removal and subtalar arthrolysis during the study period but there were no cases of secondary fusion.

In cases of significant malunion where the subtalar articular surface is displaced but intact, a joint-preserving osteotomy is the preferred procedure with the goal to restore calcaneal morphology and reduce displaced fracture components, particularly involving the posterior facet, to preinjury anatomic position. Progression of radiographic subtalar osteoarthritis is likely following corrective osteotomy but can be asymptomatic. Moreover, if subtalar degenerative disease progresses following osteotomy and symptoms preclude ongoing joint preservation, the corrected anatomy provides a more workable platform for future arthrodesis procedures.

Tips and tricks joint-preserving osteotomy

Because of the need to restore height to the hindfoot, a vertical incision is generally required, although it may be acceptable to use an oblique incision centered over the sinus tarsi if all that is required is an oblique osteotomy to restore the plane of the joint. The majority of these malunions will be associated with a varus deformity of the calcaneus with the tuberosity shifted laterally and superiorly. The first step is to identify the malunion along the plane of the original fracture using a fluoroscopic hindfoot alignment view or a modified Broden's view. It is not always possible to visualize the joint surface at this stage because the displaced lateral tuberosity will obscure the joint. A guide pin is then inserted under fluoroscopy along the precise axis of the fracture line and an osteotomy made in the exact plane of the guide pin from posterior superior to inferior and medial. Once the osteotomy is complete, it should now be easy to visualize the medial articulation and then lever the lateral tuberosity inferiorly. The tuberosity will also have to be manipulated into valgus to correct the varus malunion. A decision now has to be made as to whether an osteotomy alone will suffice or whether to combine this with a subtalar arthrodesis. If a decision has already been made to perform an arthrodesis, then following the osteotomy, the lateral wall is levered inferiorly and pinned from lateral to medial to hold the position reduced. The joint surfaces are debrided and the arthrodesis performed with fully threaded screws because compression of the joint here may not be desirable.

Subtalar Arthrodesis

Historically, subtalar arthrodesis has been the accepted treatment of advanced posttraumatic subtalar arthrosis following calcaneus fracture. Persistent pain, in the setting of mildly displaced fractures with intact calcaneal height and width treated conservatively or a displaced fracture adequately treated operatively, will predominantly be due to incongruence or cartilage damage at the subtalar joint, and these patients typically respond well to an in situ arthrodesis. Often, joint preparation and the lateral wall exostectomy can be accomplished through a limited sinus tarsi approach (**Fig. 3**). If needed, laterally placed hardware can be removed percutaneously in combination with the sinus tarsi exposure. A number of biomechanical studies have compared the optimal screw configuration for fixation of the subtalar joint in situations of isolated in situ arthrodesis.[15,16] It is well accepted that a double-divergent screw configuration achieves the greatest compression and torsional stability (**Fig. 4**). On the other side of the spectrum, severely displaced fractures treated conservatively or failed operatively treated fractures, where calcaneal height and width are not restored, will likely cause pain at the arthritic subtalar joint in addition to other deformity-driven pain generators. In these cases, some form of hindfoot realignment will be required with the subtalar arthrodesis. The most commonly used technique has been the subtalar distraction bone block arthrodesis. It is frequently necessary to combine other procedures, such as a lateral wall exostectomy, with these deformity-correcting arthrodeses as well.

Chandler and colleagues[17] retrospectively reviewed 19 cases of in situ subtalar fusions performed for the indication of late sequalae following calcaneus fractures. The authors endeavored to determine which sources of pain were and were not addressed

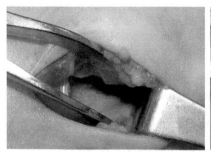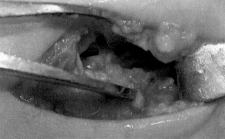

Fig. 3. The sinus tarsi exposure to the subtalar joint. Note the excellent visualization of the posterior facet. This approach can be used in the absence of significant deformity for in situ arthrodesis purposes. A lateral wall exostectomy can also be performed through this exposure. In the setting of retained orthopedic hardware from previous open reduction internal fixation, screws can be removed percutaneously in combination with this approach. The photo on the right depicts joint preparation following the removal of remaining cartilage and fish scaling using an osteotome.

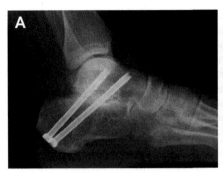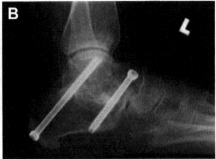

Fig. 4. Two different subtalar arthrodesis screw configurations are presented here. Inserting both screws antegrade from the heel can be technically difficult (*A*). It may be easier to insert the second screw more in retrograde fashion from the neck of the talus just lateral to the anterior tibial tendon (*B*). This screw, when placed second, can be fully threaded after compression has already been provided with the first partially threaded anterograde screw.

by the arthrodesis procedure. They found anterior ankle tenderness to be a consistent finding in all patients who remained limited in ankle dorsiflexion (<10°) following the arthrodesis. However, there was neither a correlation between the loss of ankle dorsiflexion and postoperative talar declination values nor a correlation between overall patient outcome scores and talar declination. The authors concluded that the clinical findings of anterior ankle pain and dorsiflexion restriction, rather than radiographic parameters, should guide the decision when considering distraction subtalar arthrodesis.

Tips and tricks in situ arthrodesis

When to use a small sinus tarsi incision, and when to use a more extensile incision? It is quite reasonable to use a sinus tarsi approach even if the fracture had been treated using an extensile incision because these heal very well. It is our preference to use an extensile approach to arthrodesis regardless of the original incision when there is hardware buried that cannot be easily removed percutaneously. This extensile approach facilitates the removal of all excess lateral bone, the removal of buried hardware, and, most importantly, the inspection of the peroneal tendons that may be dislocated or torn. In the event that, an ankle ligament reconstruction needs to be performed, a nonanatomic procedure can be used with half of the brevis tendon. Regardless of the approach to the arthrodesis, it is essential to remove enough bone from the lateral wall such that the lateral calcaneal shoulder is medial to the lateral wall of the talus.

Calcaneal fracture malunions with significant loss of heel height and advanced arthrosis are generally approached with the goal of reestablishing normal talar declination simultaneously with the elimination of the painful subtalar joint through arthrodesis. Restoration of ankle biomechanics is preferred in this setting to maximize limb function and limit the progression or development of tibiotalar degeneration. In order to accomplish this, a structural bone block must be placed in the position of the native subtalar joint posterior facet. Carr first published on this concept in 1988.[18] Over time, the indications for distraction arthrodesis have been refined as has the understanding of potential pitfalls associated with the surgical technique.

Myerson and Quill used a loss of heel height of more than 8 mm, compared with the opposite foot on weight-bearing lateral radiographs, as their indication to perform bone-block distraction arthrodesis for 14 patients with subtalar arthrosis in a retrospective study on the empiric management of calcaneus fracture malunions.[19] The presence or absence of anterior ankle pain and radiographic evidence of bony anterior tibiotalar impingement was noted but did not influence the choice of procedure. Seven patients (50%) reported good results and 3 (21%) fair at an average of 32 months after the arthrodesis. Two of the patients who reported poor outcomes had pain along the plantar lateral border of the foot and were found to have varus malunion at the arthrodesis site. Their scores and function were improved following corrective revision using a closing-wedge valgus calcaneal osteotomy.

In a larger series of 37 subtalar bone block arthrodeses, with the vast majority treated for the indication of calcaneus fracture sequelae, Trnka and colleagues[20] found better success rates. For those patients who went on to union (86%), AOFAS hindfoot scores improved from 21.1 preoperatively to 68.9 at a mean final follow-up of 70 months. Twenty-nine of the 31 patients who achieved union reported satisfaction with the procedure. The 2 unsatisfied patients had ongoing nerve-related syndromes. Radiological analysis showed statistically significant correction in talocalcaneal angle, calcaneal pitch, and talar declination angle between preoperative and final follow-up radiographs. Of note, comparison of initial postoperative radiographs with those at final follow-up showed a loss of correction in most radiographic parameters. The authors proposed that this finding represented hindfoot settling during graft incorporation. Similar observations in postoperative graft height loss have been reported following distraction subtalar arthrodesis.[21] There were 5 total nonunions in Trnka's series, 4 of which occurred in patients treated with femoral head allograft bone block.

The above studies introduced a number of guidelines that have influenced the evolution of this procedure. The authors recommend approaching the subtalar joint from posterolaterally via a longitudinal incision in the manner described by Gallie.[22] This is to minimize tension on the wound closure that can occur in horizontal approaches when the hindfoot is lengthened. In general, wound complications have been limited to superficial infections with rarely reported wound dehiscence when this approach is used. To avoid varus subtalar joint position a femoral distractor can be placed medially with external fixator pins in the calcaneus and tibia to impart the desired amount of valgus. Additionally, the bone block can be fashioned into a trapezoidal shape to preferentially distract more on the medial side of the subtalar joint. Subtalar arthrodesis should be supplemented with a lateral wall exostectomy when peroneal tendinitis and/or calcaneofibular impingement is present (**Fig. 5**).

Schepers performed a systematic review on the functional outcome of subtalar distraction bone block arthrodesis in the treatment of failed initial management of displaced intra-articular calcaneal fractures.[23] The review included 21 studies involving 372 cases. Overall wound complications were pooled at about 6% with an overall union rate of about 96% with most studies using tricortical iliac crest autograft for the bone block. The average modified AOFAS hindfoot score at final follow-up was 73. Six studies reported on prereconstruction and postreconstruction AOFAS hindfoot scores with an average improvement of 44.2 points.

Tips and tricks distraction bone block arthrodesis

- A vertical incision is generally necessary.
- If a lateral incision is used, then anticipate wound healing issues.
- It is ideal to retract the sural nerve posteriorly.
- Elevate the peroneal tendons with a large periosteal elevator off the lateral wall.
- Perform a generous lateral wall ostectomy going as far anteriorly as possible.
- Visualize the subtalar joint under fluoroscopy with a small curved osteotome.
- With the small osteotome in place, use a larger one to lever open the joint.

- As the joint begins to open insert a laminar spreader and gradually distract the joint.
- Check the restored talar declination angle to determine the size of the graft.
- If available, use custom trials to measure the size of the defect and graft required.
- Be very careful not to tilt the heel into varus during distraction.
- Use custom grafts if available but if not, then cut the graft higher medially than laterally to force the heel into valgus.
- Over distract to be able to insert the graft and remove the spreader.
- Use fully threaded screw(s) for fixation.

Recognizing some of the potential technical challenges associated with distraction subtalar arthrodesis, other investigators have proposed methods to correct the loss of calcaneal height without inclusion of bone block distraction by way of in situ arthrodesis combined with a vertical osteotomy and inferior slide of the calcaneal tuberosity (**Fig. 6**). Haddad has presented on his experience with this technique (referenced via direct communication). The technique aims to indirectly restore talar plantarflexion via recreation of a more elevated calcaneal pitch. Huang and colleagues[24] published on their version of this technique in 1999. They described performing the osteotomy and in situ subtalar arthrodesis through an extensile lateral approach. Autologous bone harvested from the lateral wall exostectomy was used to augment the fusion site. In cases where tension in the Achilles tendon limited the ability to inferiorly translate the calcaneal tuberosity by 1 cm (cm), a Z-lengthening was performed concomitantly. Subjective satisfaction ratings did not differ between a group of patients treated with this osteotomy and another group treated with the in situ arthrodesis without the osteotomy. Unfortunately, the interpretation of objective comparisons is limited in this study, and there is no commentary on the technique's impact on talar declination angle or ankle motion, and hence, its ability to improve ankle biomechanics and function remains largely unknown.

Other osteotomies may be necessary during arthrodesis of the subtalar joint to address other deformities (**Figs. 7** and **8**). The most commonly encountered deformity

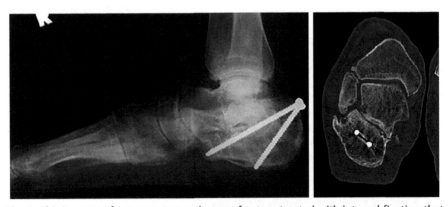

Fig. 5. This is a case of a tongue-type calcaneus fracture treated with internal fixation that developed collapse of the posterior facet with a shortened heel and painful posttraumatic subtalar arthrosis. The coronal plane CT slice also demonstrates calcaneofibular abutment secondary to healed bone from lateral wall blowout. This case of impingement will require a lateral wall decompression in addition to subtalar arthrodesis. Consideration must be given to a bone block arthrodesis as well. There is only mild axial malalignment so a simultaneous osteotomy does not need to be added to the procedure.

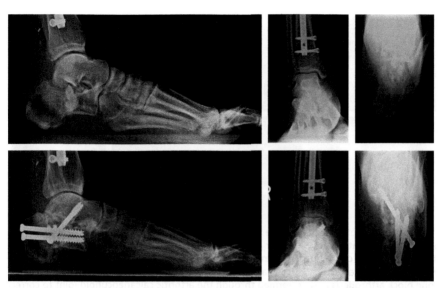

Fig. 6. This is a case where an inferior slide calcaneal tuberosity osteotomy was performed for a shortened malunion instead of a subtalar bone block arthrodesis. This patient had a good result, However, there does not seem to be a change of the talar declination angle. Case and radiographic images courtesy of Steven Haddad, MD.

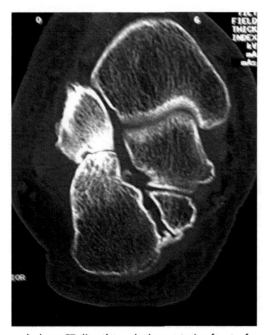

Fig. 7. This is a coronal plane CT slice through the posterior facet of a severely malunited calcaneus fracture dislocation. The lateral portion of the posterior facet is displaced laterally and superiorly and is in contact with the distal fibula leading to painful abutment syndrome. This malunion cannot be adequately treated without an osteotomy through the fracture site, in addition to a subtalar arthrodesis.

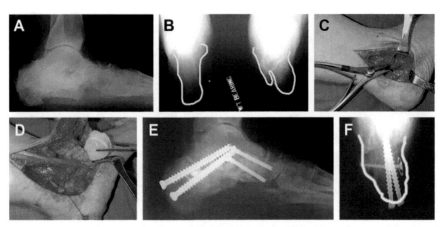

Fig. 8. This patient had undergone multiple prior surgeries with a shortened heel and nonunion of the attempted subtalar arthrodesis (*A*). Severe valgus was present (*B*) in addition to abduction of the foot with crushing of the calcaneocuboid joint. In addition to the subtalar bone block arthrodesis, a calcaneus osteotomy was performed (*C*). An additional bone block arthrodesis was performed through the arthritic calcaneocuboid joint to correct the abduction (*D*). The extensile incision used here is acceptable because the vertical height added did not place any stress on the posterior incision. Note the corrected calcaneal pitch, talar declination angle, and hindfoot coronal plane alignment (*E, F*).

is a varus malunion. Farouk and colleagues[25] performed subtalar arthrodesis, lateral wall exostectomy and lateral closing wedge calcaneal osteotomies in their prospective study involving 18 patients with Sanders type 3 calcaneal fracture malunions. At 18 months, the authors reported statistically significant improvements in patient reported outcomes including AOFAS and VAS scores. They also conducted preoperative and postoperative gait analyses and reported improvements in patient comfortable walking speed as well as maximum ground reaction force exerted during

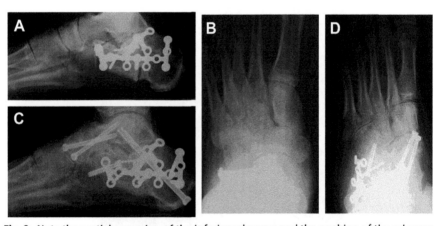

Fig. 9. Note the partial nonunion of the inferior calcaneus and the crushing of the calcaneocuboid joint. In addition, there is significant subchondral sclerosis and joint space loss involving the talonavicular articulation (*A, B*). This patient had relatively well-preserved overall calcaneal morphology. Nonetheless, the patient had significant pain in the sinus tarsi and calcaneocuboid joint. The nonunion eventually healed following revision surgery to triple arthrodesis (*C, D*).

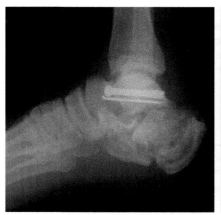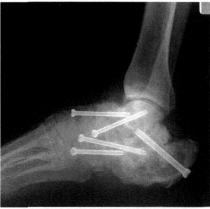

Fig. 10. Note the need for a triple arthrodesis with a bone block graft in this case. However, it must also be noted that although pain relief was achieved, the patient complained of anterior ankle impingement due to a negative talar declination angle. A revision of the procedure with a calcaneus osteotomy was recommended but refused by the patient.

the push-off phase of gait cycle. Heel valgus angle, as measured by routine CT scan at 18 months, was uniformly improved. There were no cases of nonunion.

There are situations where an extended hindfoot arthrodesis may be considered for the treatment of posttraumatic arthritis and deformity secondary to a calcaneus fracture malunion (**Figs. 9** and **10**). If possible, this should be avoided. These situations include concomitant painful arthritis involving the calcaneocuboid and/or talonavicular joints or fixed deformities through the transverse tarsal joint that cannot be amended with corrective arthrodesis through the subtalar joint. Molloy and Myerson published on the utility of triple arthrodesis specifically in the setting of symptomatic calcaneus fracture nonunion.[26] In their series of 14 intra-articular nonunions, 4 patients necessitated inclusion of the calcaneocuboid and talonavicular joints in the reconstructive fusion in order to obtain adequate fixation. Historically, results for triple arthrodesis have been poor.

SUMMARY

The management options for the painful subtalar joint following calcaneus fracture malunion are numerous. In general, the most appropriate treatment is largely dictated by the degree of concomitant residual calcaneus deformity. When calcaneus fractures are minimally displaced to begin with or undergo open reduction and internal fixation with reestablishment of close to anatomic morphology, effective management of the patient's symptoms may be limited to the subtalar joint alone. In these cases, arthroscopic or open limited debridement may be indicated. When subtalar arthritis is advanced, in situ arthrodesis is the treatment of choice. In cases of displaced malunion with relatively intact articular surfaces, joint-preserving osteotomies may be considered. Finally, in the setting of combined deformity and end-stage arthrosis, the goal of treatment will be to reconstruct calcaneal morphology with simultaneous fusion of the subtalar joint. When the predominant deformity is collapse with loss of heel height and signs of anterior ankle impingement, a distraction bone block arthrodesis is used to correct the angle of the talus. When there is an additional coronal plane deformity, such as hindfoot varus, a lateral closing wedge osteotomy is typically added. In most cases of calcaneus malunion, a lateral wall exostectomy should be added to decompress subfibular impingement and peroneal tendon irritation. As previously stated, calcaneal fracture malunions are associated with a myriad of potential symptom generators related to the most common deformities and secondary pathomechanics. A meticulous physical examination and imaging workup is paramount in identifying these pain sources and structuring an individualized treatment approach for these patients.

CLINICS CARE POINTS

- When appropriate, anatomic restoration of intra-articular calcaneus fractures is advised to reestablish bony morphology and subtalar joint biomechanics.
- When considering surgical treatment of a patient with hindfoot pain and a history of calcaneus fracture, a computed tomographic scan is essential for understanding deformity and appropriate preoperative planning.
- Patients must be evaluated for concomitant symptomatic pathologic condition such as subfibular impingement, anterior tibiotalar arthrosis, and peroneal tendon instability.
- When calcaneal morphology is well preserved but there is symptomatic focal chondromalacia or posttraumatic arthrofibrosis, joint-preserving techniques such as open or arthroscopic debridement can be used.
- When there is significant subtalar joint displacement but the posterior facet articular surfaces are healthy, recreation of the fracture through intra-articular osteotomy should be considered to restore anatomy.
- When there is advanced arthrosis involving the subtalar joint, arthrodesis should be pursued.
- For an unsalvageable subtalar joint in the setting of minimal calcaneal deformity, in situ arthrodesis is the accepted treatment.
- Distraction bone block subtalar arthrodesis should be considered when there is advanced subtalar joint disease and significant hindfoot shortening.
- When planning to restore hindfoot height through calcaneal osteotomies or through distraction bone block arthrodesis, incisions should be made longitudinally to avoid tension during closure.

DISCLOSURE

The authors have nothing to disclose.

REFERENCES

1. Rammelt S, Zwipp H. Calcaneus fractures: facts, controversies and recent developments. Injury 2004;35(5):443–61.
2. Csizy M, Buckley R, Tough S, et al. Displaced intra-articular calcaneal fractures: variables predicting late subtalar fusion. J Orthop Trauma 2003;17:106–12.
3. Mann RA, Baumgarten M. Subtalar fusion for isolated subtalar disorders. Preliminary report. Clin Orthop Relat Res 1988;(226):260–5.
4. Sanders R, Fortin P, DiPasquale T, et al. Operative treatment in 120 displaced intraarticular calcaneal fractures. Results using a prognostic computed tomography scan classification. Clin Orthop Relat Res 1993;290:87–95.
5. Heier KA, Infante AF, Walling AK, et al. Open fractures of the calcaneus: soft-tissue injury determines outcome. J Bone Joint Surg Am 2003;85(12):2276–82.

6. Stephens HM, Sanders R. Calcaneal malunions: results of a prognostic computed tomography classification system. Foot Ankle Int 1996;17(7):395–401.
7. Zwipp H, Rammelt S. Subtalar arthrodesis with calcaneal osteotomy. Orthopade 2006;35(4):387–98, 400-398.
8. Welck MJ, Myerson MS. The value of Weight-Bearing CT scan in the evaluation of subtalar distraction bone block arthrodesis: case report. Foot Ankle Surg 2015; 21(4):e55–9.
9. Elgafy H, Ebraheim NA. Subtalar arthroscopy for persistent subfibular pain after calcaneal fractures. Foot Ankle Int 1999;20(7):422–7.
10. Lee KB, Chung JY, Song EK, et al. Arthroscopic release for painful subtalar stiffness after intra-articular fractures of the calcaneum. J Bone Joint Surg Br 2008; 90(11):1457–61.
11. Kim GL, Park JY, Hyun YS, et al. Treatment of traumatic subtalar arthritis with interpositional arthroplasty with tensor fascia lata or fat. Eur J Orthop Surg Traumatol 2013;23(4):487–91.
12. Benirschke SK, Kramer PA. Joint-Preserving Osteotomies for Malaligned Intraarticular Calcaneal Fractures. Foot Ankle Clin 2016;21(1):111–22.
13. Yu GR, Hu SJ, Yang YF, et al. Reconstruction of calcaneal fracture malunion with osteotomy and subtalar joint salvage: technique and outcomes. Foot Ankle Int 2013;34(5):726–33.
14. Rammelt S, Grass R, Zwipp H. Joint-preserving osteotomy for malunited intraarticular calcaneal fractures. J Orthop Trauma 2013;27(10):e234–8.
15. Jastifer JR, Alrafeek S, Howard P, et al. Biomechanical evaluation of strength and stiffness of subtalar joint arthrodesis screw constructs. Foot Ankle Int 2016;37(4): 419–26.
16. Chuckpaiwong B, Easley ME, Glisson RR. Screw placement in subtalar arthrodesis: a biomechanical study. Foot Ankle Int 2009;30(2):133–41.
17. Chandler JT, Bonar SK, Anderson RB, et al. Results of in situ subtalar arthrodesis for late sequelae of calcaneus fractures. Foot Ankle Int 1999;20(1):18–24.
18. Carr JB, Hansen ST, Benirschke SK. Subtalar distraction bone block fusion for late complications of os calcis fractures. Foot Ankle 1988;9(2):81–6.
19. Myerson M, Quill GE Jr. Late complications of fractures of the calcaneus. J Bone Joint Surg Am 1993;75(3):331–41.
20. Trnka HJ, Easley ME, Lam PW, et al. Subtalar distraction bone block arthrodesis. J Bone Joint Surg Br 2001;83(6):849–54.
21. Chan SC, Alexander IJ. Subtalar arthrodesis with interposition tricortical iliac crest graft for late pain and deformity after calcaneus fracture. Foot Ankle Int 1997;18(10):613–5.
22. Gallie WE. Subastragalar arthrodesis in fractures of the os calcis. J Bone Joint Surg 1943;25(4):731–6.
23. Schepers T. The subtalar distraction bone block arthrodesis following the late complications of calcaneal fractures: a systematic review. Foot 2013;23(1):39–44.
24. Huang PJ, Fu YC, Cheng YM, et al. Subtalar arthrodesis for late sequelae of calcaneal fractures: fusion in situ versus fusion with sliding corrective osteotomy. Foot Ankle Int 1999;20(3):166–70.
25. Farouk A, Ibrahim A, Abd-Ella MM, et al. Effect of Subtalar fusion and calcaneal osteotomy on function, pain, and gait mechanics for calcaneal malunion. Foot Ankle Int 2019;40(9):1094–103.
26. Molloy AP, Myerson MS, Yoon P. Symptomatic nonunion after fracture of the calcaneum. Demographics and treatment. J Bone Joint Surg Br 2007;89(9): 1218–24.

Double and Triple Tarsal Fusions in the Severe Rigid Flatfoot Deformity

Naji S. Madi, MD[a],*, Amanda N. Fletcher, MD, MSc[b],
Mark E. Easley, MD[b]

KEYWORDS

- Flatfoot deformity • Triple arthrodesis • Double arthrodesis • Rigid deformity
- Malunion • Nonunion

KEY POINTS

- A rigid flatfoot deformity is characterized by dorsolateral subluxation of the navicular bone on the talus, a fixed forefoot varus, and a lateral column shortening.
- Triple arthrodesis (ST, TN, CC joints) has been the historical standard procedure to correct rigid hindfoot deformities and arthritis. Sparing the CC joint has been performed with inconsistent results.
- Dual incision has been the traditional approach for triple arthrodesis. A single medial incision could be considered in high-risk patients.
- Hindfoot valgus is usually better tolerated than overcorrection into hindfoot varus.
- A transverse tarsal osteotomy is a powerful tool that has been employed to correct different types of residual deformities.

BRIEF OVERVIEW OF THE DEFORMITY

An adult acquired flatfoot deformity, or as recently described, progressive collapsing flatfoot deformity,[1] is a multiplanar foot deformity characterized by forefoot abduction and supination and hindfoot valgus. Typically, the navicular bone rotates laterally and everts around the talar head, resulting in lateral deviation or abduction of the forefoot. Less frequently, the apex of this deformity can be at the naviculocuneiform or tarsometatarsal joints. The forefoot varus, often times described as forefoot supination, is a coronal plane deformity that results in the elevation of the first ray above the fifth

The authors disclose no conflict of interests.
a Foot & Ankle Surgery, Department of Orthopaedic Surgery, West Virginia University, Morgantown, WV, USA; b Department of Orthopaedic Surgery, Duke University Medical Center, Durham, NC 27710, USA
* Corresponding author.
E-mail address: Madi.Naji@live.com
Twitter: @NajiMady (N.S.M.)

foot.theclinics.com

ray. Lateral deviation of the calcaneus then results in a valgus hindfoot deformity with plantarflexion of the talar head. The forefoot and the cuboid follow the calcaneal deviation which leads to a further abduction deformity. These deformities can occur through one of the multiple joints.[2] The soft tissue contribution to this disorder includes loss of the medial arch support (Posterior Tibialis Tendon and/or Spring ligament pathology), medial column hypermobility, and tightness of the Achilles tendon leading to an increased valgus moment. With progressive pathology, a rigid deformity may develop characterized by dorsolateral subluxation of the navicular bone on the talus, a fixed forefoot varus, and lateral column shortening with or without arthritic changes in the hindfoot joints.

CLASSIFICATION

Recently, the consensus group proposed a new classification system and nomenclature. Rather than the historic nomenclature of "adult acquired flatfoot deformity," "progressive collapsing foot deformity (PCFD)"[1] was thought to describe more accurately the worsening nature and three-dimensional deformity of this disorder. The new classification system is based on the flexibility, type, and location of deformity. This system is based on deformities that are either flexible (Stage I) or rigid (Stage II) and further described by adding 1 or more types of present deformities (classes A–E) determined by deformity location, clinical, and radiographic findings. This article will focus on the role of tarsal arthrodesis in the setting of Stage II (rigid) PCFD.

HINDFOOT ARTHRODESIS FOR RIGID DEFORMITY

The apex of rigid PCFD deformities is commonly seen at the talonavicular (TN) joint. In a cadaveric model of simulated TN joint arthrodesis, the motion in the subtalar (ST) and calcaneocuboid (CC) joints was severely limited.[3,4] The ST joint arthrodesis limited 74% and 44% of the TN and CC joints motion, respectively. The CC joint arthrodesis had minimal effect on the ST joint but restricted 33% of the TN joint motion. In a flexible (Stage I) deformity, both soft tissue balancing procedures and bony arthrodesis may be performed based on the severity of the deformity, patient factors, and surgeon preference. Which and how many joints to fuse has been debated. Harper and colleagues reported successful correction of the foot position with single TN joint arthrodesis while other authors support multiple joint arthrodesis.

In the setting of a rigid (Stage II) deformity, the appropriate procedure to use is not without controversy. The extent of joints involved in the arthrodesis depends on the ability to obtain a plantigrade foot. Both double and triple arthrodesis have been suggested. Triple arthrodesis (ST, TN, CC joints) has been the historical gold standard procedure to correct rigid hindfoot deformities and arthritis. To achieve adequate coronal plane correction (hindfoot valgus deformity), the ST joint must be fused in addition to the TN joint for the correction of the forefoot supination and abduction. Sparing the CC joint in a double arthrodesis has been performed less commonly and with inconsistent results.[5]

DOUBLE OR TRIPLE ARTHRODESIS

There is no level 1 evidence comparing double versus triple arthrodesis for the management of PCFD. The majority of the studies are retrospective case series. Advocates for triple arthrodesis believe that superior deformity correction is achieved and that the CC joint is eliminated as a pain generator. Advocates for double arthrodesis argue that preserving the CC joint allows for retained accommodation, decreased stress, and subsequent arthritis of the surrounding joints, eliminates the need for additional lateral incisions, decreased operative time, decreased cost, and similar radiographic and clinical outcomes. Situations, where the CC joint must be included in the fusion mass, include tenderness over the CC joint, advanced CC joint arthritic changes, CC joint subluxation, and inability to achieve adequate correction intraoperatively without including the CC joint.

There have been multiple studies demonstrating comparable correction achieved by double compared to triple arthrodesis.[6,7] Sammarco used radiographic parameters to assess the completeness of deformity correction. In their series of double arthrodesis, the anteroposterior talo-second metatarsal angle (forefoot abduction), the lateral talo-second metatarsal angle (arch alignment), and the lateral talocalcaneal angle improved to a range comparable to triple arthrodesis.

Normal ambulation requires a flexible foot, and, thus, any hindfoot arthrodesis procedure results in altered plantar pressure distribution and increased loading forces on adjacent joints. Preserving the CC joint can provide more movement and decrease the stress on surrounding joints.[8] Additionally, it has been demonstrated that preserving minimal motion across the CC joint allows for retained accommodation on uneven surfaces[9] and that the nonfused CC joint may adapt with time to allow more motion.

Smith and colleagues[10] reported on 27 patients who had undergone a triple arthrodesis at an average follow-up of fourteen years. While there was an overall satisfaction rate of 93%, 74% of patients reported moderate to severe difficulty with uneven surfaces and only 42% could perform a moderate activity with mild or no pain. The prevalence of severe arthritic changes was common in this series including 7 (27%) tibiotalar joints, 7 (27%) naviculocuneiform joints, and 6 (23%) tarsometatarsal joints. In a series of 77 patients at an average 15-month follow-up, Hyer and colleagues[11] reported higher odds of an increased rate of tibiotalar valgus in the triple group as compared to the double arthrodesis group. These findings suggest increased pathology to the surrounding joints following triple compared to double arthrodesis.

In a prospective comparative study of 2 cohorts undergoing double versus triple arthrodesis for adult-acquired flatfoot deformity due to stage III posterior tibial tendon insufficiency, Fadle and colleagues[6] reported double arthrodesis is an equally reliable surgical option for achieving union, improving the functional outcomes, and deformity correction as triple arthrodesis. Given the similar outcomes yet significantly shorter operative time, the authors of reference recommend double arthrodesis if the calcaneocuboid joint is unaffected.[6] In addition to shorter operative time, double arthrodesis is associated with a lower overall cost due to requiring fewer implants. Triple arthrodesis implants had an average of 2.4 times the cost as those required for double arthrodesis.[12] Additionally, typical triple arthrodesis requires one medial and one lateral incision. Although the reported risk of lateral wound breakdown with triple arthrodesis is low,[13] double arthrodesis is often performed through a single medial incision and eliminates this risk. Lastly, preparing the CC joint avoids potential nonunion problems with this joint.

DISTRACTION ARTHRODESIS OF THE CALCANEOCUBOID JOINT

Correction of the forefoot abduction deformity through the TN joint may result in CC joint gaping, termed arthrodiastasis. In double arthrodesis, joint distraction could lead to improvement in the CC arthritis with subchondral remodeling similar to ankle distraction phenomena.[14] In triple arthrodesis, axial compression through the CC joint is required to achieve union. Care must be taken to avoid lateral column shortening and loss of foot reduction when fusing the CC joint. This calls into question the need for wedge grafting in the CC joint (distraction arthrodesis).

BONE GRAFT

Multiple graft options are available to be used in foot and ankle arthrodesis surgery including autograft, allograft, bone graft substitutes, and orthobiologics. Iliac crest autograft has been the historic gold standard option. Other sources of autograft with less donor site morbidity have been used (calcaneus, proximal or distal tibia);[15] however, the yield of osteogenic and angiogenic cells from these sites has been shown to be inferior to an iliac crest harvest.[16] Autograft can be harvested as cancellous, cortical or bone marrow aspirate. The quality of the harvest depends on the host biology and donor location. The limitations of autograft include donor site morbidity, possible limited quantity and quality, and increased operative time. Allografts are available in different shapes and forms. Demineralized bone matrix graft has been shown to promote fusion in hindfoot arthrodesis with similar union rates as iliac crest bone graft.[17]

The necessity of bone grafting has been controversial with reports showing similar union rates in primary triple arthrodesis without supplementary bone grafting to those with bone grafting.[18] However, the treatment of nonunion in foot and ankle arthrodesis is challenging. Every means to decrease this risk should be entertained. The use of allograft and orthobiologics is a low-risk addition to a triple or double arthrodesis. However, care must be taken to ensure meticulous joint(s) preparation and avoiding joint(s) distraction as a large interfragmentary gap has been shown to affect bone healing.[19]

The use of bone graft or other augmentation in a double or triple arthrodesis is at the discretion of the surgeon based on operative technique and patient biology including age and comorbidities. A combination of growth factor-enhanced bone graft with cancellous chips may be considered in high-risk patients. Filling voids may help promote fusion at the arthrodesis site. Typically, in descending order of quantity, bone graft is placed into the ST joint, TN, and then the CC joint. It is preferable to morselize the cancellous chips with a rongeur as axial compression and bony apposition should not be blocked by the bone graft chips.

SURGICAL APPROACH

The traditional triple arthrodesis is performed using 2 incisions (**Fig. 1**). One on the medial side to prepare the TN joint (in some modifications, a dorsal approach has been used) and one on the lateral hindfoot to prepare the ST and CC joints. The concerns about lateral skin breakdown, especially in the setting of severe valgus deformity, led some surgeons to describe a single medial incision for a triple[20] or modified double arthrodesis.[21]

Dual Incision

In the traditional dual-incision triple arthrodesis, the patient is placed in a modified lateral decubitus position on a beanbag.[22] A thigh tourniquet is recommended rather than a calf tourniquet given an Achilles tendon lengthening is commonly performed first. The lateral incision is made from the tip of the fibula toward the base of the fourth metatarsal. Laterally, care should be taken to protect the sural nerve and to elevate the extensor digitorum brevis muscle and fascia as one thick layer for later closure. The ST joint is distracted using a Hintermann retractor or smooth lamina spreader, and all 3 facets of the ST joint should be included in the joint preparation. Meticulous joint preparation is essential to achieve union. In all joints, use an elevator, chisel, or burr to denude all cartilage; care should be taken to preserve the subchondral bone architecture. The joint should then be irrigated to remove all cartilage debris. A drill is then used

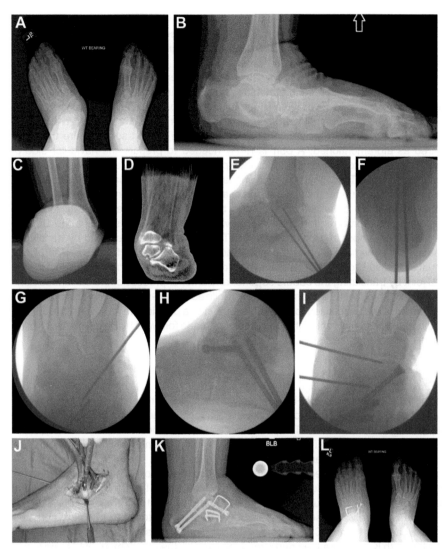

Fig. 1. 66-year-old female patient with severe pesplanovalgus deformity/peritalar dislocation. (*A*) Weightbearing Anteroposterior (AP) views of both feet. Note the severe abduction
deformity through the talonavicular joint. (*B*) Weightbearing lateral view of the left foot
showing severe arch collapse/flatfoot deformity. (*C*) Saltzman view shows a severe valgus
hindfoot deformity. (*D*) A coronal CT scan view shows the hindfoot valgus deviation and
subfibular impingement. (*E, F*) The subtalar, talonavicular (TN) and calcaneocuboid (CC)
joints were well prepped. The hindfoot valgus deformity was corrected, and a provisional
fixation was used. (*G*) The midfoot abduction and rotational deformity were corrected
then a provisional fixation across the TN joint was applied. (*H*) Definitive fixation of the subtalar and TN joints. (*I, J*) Bone block distraction, using a bone wedge, was inserted at the CC
joint and fixed with 2 staples. (*K, L*) Weightbearing AP and lateral foot views at 9-months
follow-up showing healed triple arthrodesis with the well aligned plantigrade foot.

to penetrate the subchondral bone across all facets with the drill holes about 2 mm apart. Next or concomitantly, the CC joint is prepared. A periosteal elevator can be used to release the ST joint medially. Always prepare the lateral talonavicular joint through this approach.

The dorsomedial incision is then made from the anterior medial malleolus toward the dorsomedial base of the first metatarsal. The tibialis anterior tendon should be identified and protected. In severe PCFD, the talar head bone is often weak subsequent to being uncovered; care should be taken when preparing the talar head to preserve its architecture and avoid unintentional bony removal. The joint surfaces are then prepared as aforementioned. A burr is rarely needed to prepare the navicular side of the TN joint. If indicated, bone graft is then placed at this time. Manual reduction starts with the ST joint. Through the medial and lateral incisions, you can feel the calcaneus properly reduced under the talus. A sign of an adequate reduction is the recreation of a gap between the anterolateral talus and the anterior calcaneal process. In severe cases, slight overcorrection is advised. Two retrograde K-wires across the ST joint are used for temporary fixation. Next, the TN joint is manually reduced by translating the navicular medially to cover the talar head. Provisional K-wire fixation of the TN joint must start distal against the medial aspect of the medial cuneiform. Finally, reduce the CC joint by translating the cuboid superior and anterior process of the calcaneus bone inferior. All three joints are provisionally stabilized with K-wire fixation and the overall alignment is then accessed for the achievement of a plantigrade foot. Both clinical and radiographic assessment of the correction are made followed by compression and fixation of the arthrodesis sites.

Single-Incision

In the later described single-incision approach, a single medial incision is made just posterior to the medial malleolus to the distal aspect of the navicular bone, paralleling the posterior tibialis tendon. The posterior tibial tendon sheath is opened and typically the tendon is preserved. The capsule of the TN joint is opened to expose the joint. The capsule and the tendon are peeled off of the talus and the navicular to expose the ST joint. Smooth lamina spreaders and/or Hintermann retractors are used to distract and prepare the joints. Exposure to the CC joint is challenging through this approach, and access is achieved through the TN joint. Through the lateral TN joint, the CC joint capsule is sharply released. The TN joint is then distracted with a lamina spreader to allow access to the CC joint for joint preparation. Manual reduction and provisional fixation with K-wires are then performed followed by the assessment of the correction and final fixation.

Reports have demonstrated the effectiveness of the single approach in achieving union and correcting the deformity,[23] but controversial results are reported in terms of patient satisfaction rate.[21,24] A postoperative valgus ankle deformity has been reported to develop which may be consequent of deltoid ligament damage and laxity during the ST joint approach.[12,21] In a cadaveric study, MacDonald and colleagues[25] found less cartilage denuded at the posterior facet of the ST joint and the talar head with increased tibiotalar valgus tilt in the single medial approach as compared to dual incisions.

This approach may be considered in high-risk patients with compromised, scarred, or deficient lateral soft tissues or in those with severe deformity to avoid lateral wound problems. Finally, minimally invasive techniques for a modified double arthrodesis are showing early promising results for patients at risk of wound complications.[26]

IMPLANT SELECTION

Implant selection is essential to achieve solid stabilization of the arthrodesis sites. While multiple fixation methods have been proposed for the different arthrodesis sites, there is minimal evidence supporting any particular fixation method. In a biomechanical cadaveric model of triple arthrodesis, Meyer and colleagues[27] found no difference in strength to failure between staples and screw fixation when one cannulated screw versus two staples per joint was used.

Subtalar Joint

Multiple fixation methods have been proposed for ST arthrodesis. Biomechanical cadaveric studies support the use of a 2 divergent screw construct over a single posterior screw.[28,29]

Calcaneocuboid Joint

The literature supports different constructs for CC joint fixation including screws, staples, or plate and screws. Hansen recommends 2 screws construct given the soft bone consequent to the valgus deformity.[30] Coughlin and colleagues[31] recommends multiple staples for fixation in patients with osteopenic. Kann and colleagues described an oblique single screw fixation over an axial trajectory.[32] In a cadaveric study, Milshteyn and colleagues[33] reported greater stiffness achieved with a locking compression plate compared to a 6.5 mm cancellous lag screw.

Talonavicular Joint

TN joint fixation typically includes 1 to 3 retrograde compression screws, plate and screw fixation, or staples. A combination of these has also been employed. Jarrell and colleagues[34] found no difference in with the lateralization of plantar pressure between plate and screw versus a 3 screws construct following TN joint fixation. Kiesau and colleagues[35] recommend the use of a third fully threaded screw (in addition to 2 partially threaded screws across the TN joint) from the lateral navicular into the calcaneus to decrease angulation and increase bending stiffness across the TN joint. The use of nickel–titanium alloy (Nitinol) staples is becoming more popular in foot surgery.[36] These staples are preloaded on their applicator and activated once inserted into the bone and released from the applicator; thus, the legs allow bone compression. In an in vitro study, double (perpendicular) staple constructs showed significantly higher stiffness and larger loads before 2 mm gap formation occur compared to plate fixation in all planes except ventro-dorsal and lateral right to left loading planes.[37] It is reasonable to consider using two 7.0 mm headless, fully threaded minimally divergent screws for ST joint fixation, two 5.5 mm headless screws with one Nitinol staple for the TN joint, and one 5.5 mm oblique screw from the anterior calcaneus process to the cuboid bone with or without an additional staple. Alternatively, 2 Nitinol staples may be used across the CC joint. In cases with a large navicular bone, a larger diameter (7.0 mm) screw could be used.

FAILED HINDFOOT ARTHRODESIS

The rate of nonunion following triple arthrodesis has decreased over time due to improved internal fixation and biologic augmentation techniques, with successful union rates now reported up to 95%.[18,38,39] However, deformity recurrence and malunion (undercorrection or overcorrection) rates have remained unchanged and are challenging to treat.

Malunion

Equinovarus is the most common deformity in a malunited triple arthrodesis.[40] To decrease the risk of overcorrection and malunion, the surgeon should be familiar with the hindfoot biomechanics and generate, based on the clinical examination and imaging, a meticulous preoperative plan to address and balance both the soft tissue (Achilles tendon, peroneal tendons) and bony deformity.[41]

Hindfoot valgus is usually better tolerated than overcorrection into hindfoot varus; however, undercorrection leads to subfibular impingement pain and a valgus load on the ankle (**Fig. 2**). A detailed physical examination is essential to assess the hindfoot deformity, the position of the midfoot and forefoot, previous surgical incisions, and callus formation. Radiographic assessment includes weight-bearing radiographs of the foot and ankle including an axial calcaneal view. Weight-bearing computed tomography (CT) scans are becoming increasingly available and allow a detailed understanding of the deformity and assessment of the fusion mass. Typically, undercorrection of the hindfoot valgus can be addressed with a medial displacement calcaneal osteotomy (8 to 10 mm of medial translation) with or without the removal of the previous hardware.

A hindfoot varus deformity (overcorrection) typically presents with a midfoot and forefoot deformity. In the setting of isolated hindfoot varus, a lateral closing wedge or Malerba calcaneal osteotomy could be used for deformity correction. Cody and colleagues[42] found that regardless of the osteotomy type, a lateralizing calcaneal osteotomy led to a decreased tarsal tunnel volume, hence these osteotomies must be performed with care. In the setting of severe hindfoot varus with residual forefoot supination, a combined closing wedge osteotomy through the ST joint and a rotational transverse tarsal osteotomy should be considered.

Transverse Tarsal Osteotomy

A transverse tarsal osteotomy is a powerful tool that has been employed to correct different types of deformities. In residual isolated forefoot supination or pronation, this can be performed as a rotational osteotomy. In an isolated midfoot abduction or adduction deformity, the osteotomy is performed as a medial or lateral closing wedge osteotomy, respectively. Failure to superiorly translate the cuboid at the index triple arthrodesis can lead to a rocker bottom deformity with plantar subluxation of the cuboid. This deformity may also be addressed with a plantar closing wedge transverse tarsal osteotomy. Careful attention must be paid to maintain enough navicular and cuboid bone distal to the osteotomy. In a malunited triple arthrodesis, it is not uncommon to face a combination of these deformities. A biplanar transverse tarsal osteotomy with a hindfoot osteotomy may be considered. As a rule, the correction should be performed from proximal to distal (**Fig. 3**).

Nonunion

Any joint arthrodesis has an inherent risk of nonunion. In the context of double/triple arthrodesis, while nonunion of the ST joint is a relatively rare, nonunion and delayed union of the TN joint and CC joints are more common and challenging to treat. The TN joint continues to have the highest risk of nonunion in hindfoot arthrodesis. Besides the host biology and compliance, the forces across the joint, shape of the joint, and demanding exposure for adequate joint preparation contribute to the increased risk of TN joint nonunion.

The nonunion rate of triple arthrodesis in the 1960s ranged between 10 and 23%.[43] The nonunion rate has decreased to a current range of 0 to 5%[18,38,39] which is

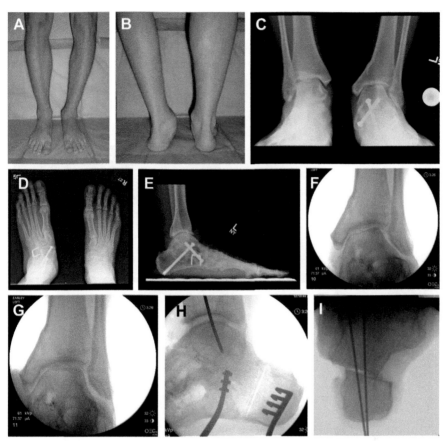

Fig. 2. 38-year-old male pharmacist with left hindfoot painful malunion S/P triple arthrodesis. (*A, B*) Clinical pictures showing the collapsed and deformed left foot and ankle. (*C*) Weight-bearing anteroposterior (AP) view of both ankles. Note the left ankle valgus deformity. (*D*) Weightbearing AP view of both feet. Note the left foot abduction deformity. (*E*) Lateral ankle view showing the healed previous triple arthrodesis with hardware in place. (*F, G*) Intraoperative fluoroscopy images showing a passively correctable valgus ankle deformity. The hardware was removed and a peroneus brevis to longus transfer was performed. (*H, I*) The ankle was pinned in a reduced position. A medial displacement calcaneal osteotomy (MDCO) was performed, and 2 pins were used for provisional fixation. (*J, K*) Intraoperative fluoroscopy AP and lateral views showing 2 wires used to mark the midfoot osteotomy. (*L*) A midfoot/hindfoot derotational osteotomy was performed using a saw. (*M*) The midfoot osteotomy was closed, and two wires were used for provisional fixation. (*N*) Final Intraoperative valgus stress view showing a stable ankle. (*O, P, Q*) Weightbearing radiographs at 1-year follow-up showing well-healed osteotomy and adequate hindfoot malunion correction. (*R*) A clinical picture at 1 year follow up showing well aligned left foot and ankle.

attributed to better internal fixation techniques and biologic augmentation.[39] There are similarly low nonunion rates reported after double arthrodesis. Sammarco and colleagues[7] reported a 94% union rate in a retrospective review of 14 patients treated with double arthrodesis for symptomatic flatfoot at an average 40-month follow-up. In the only prospective cohort reported in the literature, both double and triple arthrodesis afforded a 100% union rate with no difference in time to union.[6]

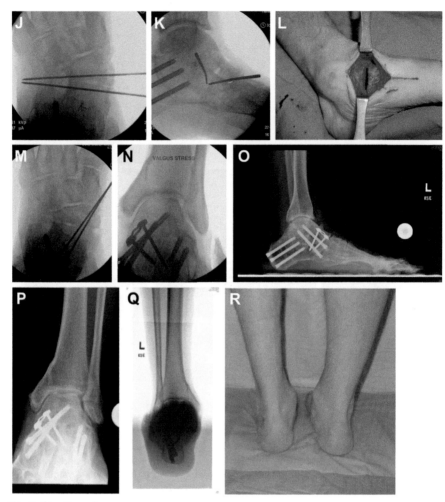

Fig. 2. (*continued*).

Upon initial assessment of a nonunited double or triple arthrodesis, an extensive review of the patient's medical history and surgical technique should be performed to determine potential factors for failure. Typically, the etiology is multifactorial. The exam should include a vascular assessment for foot perfusion. A septic nonunion must be ruled out with an inflammatory laboratory work-up (white blood cell (WBC) count, C-reactive protein, erythrocyte sedimentation rate) and advanced imaging (WBC-labeled bone scans, MRI). CT scans afford improved evaluation of bone healing compared to plain radiographs.[44]

In their report on isolated ST arthrodesis, Easley and colleagues[45] reported that, among other factors, clinically important avascularity (defined as at least 2 mm of non-bleeding subchondral bone) was associated with an increased risk of nonunion. Intraoperative recognition of avascularity at the arthrodesis sites may be an indication to add additional biologic augmentation to the arthrodesis sites to promote union. In the revision arthrodesis setting, the use of rigid internal fixation, bone graft, and other

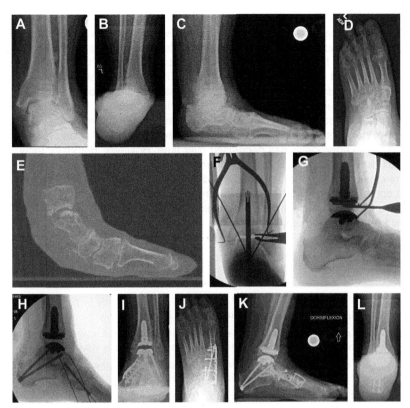

Fig. 3. 75-year-old male patient with left ankle and foot pain that failed to improve with conservative management. (*A*) Weightbearing (AP) view of the left ankle showing advanced ankle arthritis with valgus deformity. (*B*) Saltzman view showing hindfoot valgus deformity. (*C, D*) Weightbearing AP and lateral foot views showing midfoot collapse and arthritis. (*E*) Sagittal weight-bearing CT scan showing collapsed arch with arthritic changes involving the talonavicular (TN), Naviculocuneiform (NC), and first tarsometatarsal joint (TMT). (*F, G*) The ankle deformity was corrected followed by a stemmed total ankle arthroplasty (Inbone II). (*H*) The peroneal tendons were released, the hindfoot and medial column joints were prepped for arthrodesis then the foot deformity was corrected. Provisional fixation was applied. Radiographs at 5-months follow-up (*I*) AP ankle view, (*J*) AP foot view, (*K*) lateral ankle view, and (*L*) Saltzman view, showing well aligned total ankle arthroplasty and adequate correction of the foot collapse through hindfoot and medial column arthrodesis. Note the calcaneocuboid joint was not fused.

orthobiologics are critical to achieve bone healing. DiGiovanni and colleagues[46] reported that graft material filling of more than 50% of the arthrodesis site at 9 weeks was associated with higher union rates in the hindfoot and ankle at 24 weeks postoperative. We recommend the use of iliac crest cancellous graft with bone graft substitutes in the setting of revision arthrodesis.

SUMMARY

A flatfoot deformity is a multiplanar foot deformity characterized by forefoot abduction and supination and hindfoot valgus. Soft tissue contribution includes the medial structures, medial column hypermobility, and Achilles tendon tightness. The deformity could occur through multiple joints. Typically, the navicular bone rotates laterally and everts around the talar head, resulting in lateral deviation or abduction of the forefoot. Multiple classification systems have been used. Recently progressive collapsing foot deformity (PCFD) has been introduced. The apex of rigid PCFD deformities is commonly seen at the talonavicular (TN) joint. The extent of joints involved in the arthrodesis depends on the ability to obtain a plantigrade foot. Both double and triple arthrodesis have been suggested. A dual or single incisions could be used. While multiple fixation methods have been proposed for the different arthrodesis site, there is minimal evidence supporting any particular fixation method. The rate of nonunion following triple arthrodesis has decreased over time. However, deformity recurrence and malunion (undercorrection or overcorrection) rates have remained unchanged and are challenging to treat. In a malunited triple arthrodesis, it is not uncommon to face a combination of deformities. The surgeon should be familiar with the hindfoot biomechanics to decrease the risk of malunion. As a rule, the correction should be performed from proximal to distal.

CLINICS CARE POINTS

- The TN joint is commonly the apex of a PCFD.
- Double or Triple hindfoot arthrodesis could be used in a rigid PCFD.
- The rate of nonunion following triple arthrodesis has decreased over time. Deformity recurrence and malunion remain unchanged and are challenging to treat.
- The surgeon should pay a careful attention, intraoperatively, to the deformity reduction clinically and radiographically. It is crucial to avoid an over or undercorrection.
- Upon evaluation of a hindfoot nonunion, an infectious work up is recommended to rule out a septic nonunion
- Calcaneal osteotomies are a powerful tool to correct a hindfoot malunion. A transverse tarsal osteotomy could be used to correct a rotational malunion deformity.

REFERENCES

1. Myerson MS, Thordarson DB, Johnson JE, et al. Classification and nomenclature: progressive collapsing foot deformity. Foot Ankle Int 2020;41(10):1271–6.
2. Van Boerum DH, Sangeorzan BJ. Biomechanics and pathophysiology of flat foot. Foot Ankle Clin 2003;8(3):419–30.
3. Astion Donna J, Deland Jonathan T, Otis James C, Kenneally Sharon BS. Motion of the hindfoot after simulated arthrodesis. NEW YORK, N.Y. J Bone Joint Surg 1997;79(2):241–6.
4. Harper MC, Tisdel CL. Talonavicular arthrodesis for the painful adult acquired flatfoot. Foot Ankle Int 1996;17(11):658–61.
5. Burrus MT, Werner BC, Carr JB, et al. Increased failure rate of modified double arthrodesis compared with triple arthrodesis for rigid pes planovalgus. J Foot Ankle Surg 2016;55(6):1169–74.
6. Fadle AA, El-Adly W, Attia AK, et al. Double versus triple arthrodesis for adult-acquired flatfoot deformity due to stage III posterior tibial tendon insufficiency: a prospective comparative study of two cohorts. Int Orthop 2021. https://doi.org/10.1007/s00264-021-05041-1.

7. Sammarco VJ, Magur EG, Sammarco GJ, et al. Arthrodesis of the subtalar and talonavicular joints for correction of symptomatic hindfoot malalignment. Foot Ankle Int 2006;27(9):661–6.

8. Schuh R, Salzberger F, Wanivenhaus AH, et al. Kinematic changes in patients with double arthrodesis of the hindfoot for realignment of planovalgus deformity. J Orthop Res 2013;31(4):517–24.

9. Wülker N, Stukenborg C, Savory KM, et al. Hindfoot motion after isolated and combined arthrodeses: measurements in anatomic specimens. Foot Ankle Int 2000;21(11):921–7.

10. Smith RW, Shen W, DeWitt S, et al. Triple arthrodesis in adults with non-paralytic disease. J Bone Joint Surg 2004;86(12):2707–13.

11. Hyer CF, Galli MM, Scott RT, et al. Ankle valgus after hindfoot arthrodesis: a radiographic and chart comparison of the medial double and triple arthrodeses. J Foot Ankle Surg 2014;53(1):55–8.

12. Galli MM, Scott RT, Bussewitz BW, et al. A retrospective comparison of cost and efficiency of the medial double and dual incision triple arthrodeses. Foot Ankle Spec 2014;7:32–6.

13. Saltzman CL, Fehrle MJ, Cooper RR, et al. Triple arthrodesis: twenty-five and forty-four-year average follow-up of the same patients. J Bone Joint Surg Am 1999;81(10):1391–402.

14. Berlet GC, Hyer CF, Scott RT, et al. Medial double arthrodesis with lateral column sparing and arthrodiastasis: a radiographic and medical record review. J Foot Ankle Surg 2015;54(3):441–4.

15. Raikin SM, Brislin K. Local bone graft harvested from the distal tibia or calcaneus for surgery of the foot and ankle. Foot Ankle Int 2005;26(6):449–53.

16. Hyer CF, Berlet GC, Bussewitz BW. Quantitative assessment of the yield of osteoblastic connective tissue progenitors in bone marrow aspirate from the iliac crest, tibia, and calcaneus. J Bone Joint Surg Am 2013;95(14):1312–6.

17. Michelson JD, Curl LA. Use of demineralized bone matrix in hindfoot arthrodesis. Clin Orthop Relat Res 1996;325:203–8.

18. Rosenfeld PF, Budgen SA, Saxby TS. Triple arthrodesis: is bone grafting necessary? The results in 100 consecutive cases. J Bone Joint Surg Br 2005;87(2):175–8.

19. Claes L, Augat P, Suger G. Influence of size and stability of the osteotomy gap on the success of fracture healing. J Orthop Res 1997;15(4):577–84.

20. Vora A, Myerson M, Jeng C. The Medial approach to triple arthrodesis: indications and technique for management of rigid valgus deformities in high-risk patients. Tech Foot Ankle Surg 2005;4(4):258–62.

21. Anand P, Nunley JA, DeOrio JK. Single-incision medial approach for double arthrodesis of hindfoot in posterior tibialis tendon dysfunction. Foot Ankle Int 2013;34(3):338–44.

22. Easley ME. Operative techniques in foot and ankle surgery. Available from: Wolters Kluwer. 2nd edition. Philadelphia, PA: Wolters Kluwer Health; 2016.

23. Brilhault J. Single Medial Approach to modified double arthrodesis in rigid flatfoot with lateral deficient skin. Foot Ankle Int 2009;30(1):21–6.

24. Knupp M, Schuh R, Stufkens SA, et al. Subtalar and talonavicular arthrodesis through a single medial approach for the correction of severe planovalgus deformity. J Bone Joint Surg Br 2009;91:612–5.

25. MacDonald A, Anderson M, Soin S, et al. Single medial vs 2-incision approach for double hindfoot arthrodesis: is there a difference in joint preparation? Foot Ankle Int 2021;42(8):1068–73.

26. Tejero S, Carranza-Pérez-Tinao A, Zambrano-Jiménez MD, et al. Minimally invasive technique for stage III adult-acquired flatfoot deformity: a mid- to long-term retrospective study. Int Orthopaedics 2021;45:217–23 (SICOT).

27. Meyer MS, Alvarez BE, Njus GO, et al. Triple arthrodesis: a biomechanical evaluation of screw versus staple fixation. Foot Ankle Int 1996;17(12):764–7.

28. Chuckpaiwong B, Easley ME, Glisson RR. Screw placement in subtalar arthrodesis: a biomechanical study. Foot Ankle Int 2009;30(2):133–41.

29. Jastifer JR, Alrafeek S, Howard P, et al. Biomechanical evaluation of strength and stiffness of subtalar joint arthrodesis screw constructs. Foot Ankle Int 2016;37(4):419–26.

30. Hansen ST. Functional reconstruction of the foot and ankle. Philadelphia, PA: Lippincott Williams & Wilkins; 2000.

31. Coughlin MJ, Mann RA, Saltzman C. Surgery of the foot and ankle. 8th ed. Philadelphia, PA: Mosby Elsevier; 2007.

32. Kann JN, Parks BG, Schon LC. Biomechanical evaluation of two different screw positions for fusion of the calcaneocuboid joint. Foot Ankle Int 1999;20(1):33–6.

33. Milshteyn MA, Dwyer M, Andrecovich C, et al. Comparison of two fixation methods for arthrodesis of the calcaneocuboid joint: a biomechanical study. Foot Ankle Int 2015;36(1):98–102.

34. Jarrell SE, Owen JR, Wayne JS, et al. Biomechanical comparison of screw versus plate/screw construct for talonavicular fusion. Foot Ankle Int 2009;30(2):150–6.

35. Kiesau CD, LaRose CR, Glisson RR, et al. Talonavicular joint fixation using augmenting naviculocalcaneal screw in modified double hindfoot arthrodesis. Foot Ankle Int 2011;32(3):244–9.

36. Malal JG, Kumar CS. The use of memory® staples in foot and ankle surgery. Br Orthopaedic Foot Surg Soc 2018;90(B). https://doi.org/10.1302/0301-620X.90BSUPP_II.0900231.

37. Hoon QJ, Pelletier MH, Christou C, et al. Biomechanical evaluation of shape-memory alloy staples for internal fixation-an in vitro study. J Exp Orthop 2016;3(1):19.

38. Pell R 4th, Myerson MS, Schon IC. Clinical outcome after primary triple arthrodesis. J Bone Joint Surg Am 2000;82-A:47–57.

39. Bednarz PA, Monroe MT, Manoli A. Triple arthrodesis in adults using rigid internal fixation: an assessment of outcome. Foot Ankle Int 1999;20(6):356–63.

40. Bibbo C, Anderson RB, Davis WH. Complications of midfoot and hindfoot arthrodesis. Clin Orthop Relat Res 2001;391:45–58.

41. Seybold JD. Management of the Malunited Triple Arthrodesis. Foot Ankle Clin 2017;22(3):625–36.

42. Cody EA, Greditzer HG, MacMahon A, et al. Effects on the tarsal tunnel following malerba Z-type osteotomy compared to standard lateralizing calcaneal osteotomy. Foot Ankle Int 2016;37(9):1017–22.

43. Wilson F, Fay G, Lamotte P, et al. Triple arthrodesis: a study of factors affecting fusion after three hundred and one procedures. J Bone Joint Surg Am 1965;47-A:340–8.

44. Jones CP, Coughlin MJ, Shurnas PS. Prospective CT scan evaluation of hindfoot nonunions treated with revision surgery and low-intensity ultrasound stimulation. Foot Ankle Int 2006;27(4):229–35.

45. Easley ME, Trnka H, Schon LC, et al. Isolated subtalar arthrodesis. J Bone Joint Surg 2000;82(5):613.

46. DiGiovanni CW, Lin SS, Daniels TR, et al. The importance of sufficient graft material in achieving foot or ankle fusion. J Bone Joint Surg Am 2016;98(15):1260–7.

Double and Triple Tarsal Fusions in the Complex Cavovarus Foot

Wolfram Wenz, MD

KEYWORDS

- Cavovarus foot deformity • Surgical correction • Tendon transfer • Arthrodesis
- Double fusion • Triple tarsal fusions

KEY POINTS

- Always start correcting at the hindfoot not with the forefoot.
- Tendon transfers are mandatory in every case.
- A foot will deform in the presence of a solid, well-performed triple arthrodesis when the foot is not in gross muscular balance.

INTRODUCTION

Cavus foot is characterized by increased plantar flexion of the forefoot and midfoot in relation to the hindfoot resulting in high foot arch. Because cavus foot rarely occurs in an isolated form, the term "cavus foot" rather describes a part of a complex multiplanar foot deformity, which is commonly accompanied by various components in other planes.

Basically, 4 different types of cavus deformity are commonly described: the "pure" cavus foot (**Fig. 1**A), the cavovarus foot (**Fig. 1**B), the equinocavovarus foot (**Fig. 1**C), and the calcaneocavus foot (**Fig. 1**D), which may present with additional hindfoot valgus or varus deformity.

The different types of cavus deformity may be distinguished by their cause, pathogenesis, as well as clinical and radiographic appearances. **Table 1** summarizes the characteristics of the 4 types of cavus deformity.

UNDERSTANDING THE DEFORMITY

Understanding the underlying pathologic condition is essential for a successful deformity correction. For the cavus foot this may be a challenge because various causes may be responsible for the development of the deformity. It is therefore important

EXPERTS FIRST Die Knochen-Docs, Rudolf-Diesel-Straße 11, Heidelberg 69115, Germany
E-mail address: wenz@experts-first.de
Website: http://www.experts-first.de

Foot Ankle Clin N Am 27 (2022) 819–833
https://doi.org/10.1016/j.fcl.2022.08.004
1083-7515/22/© 2022 Elsevier Inc. All rights reserved.

foot.theclinics.com

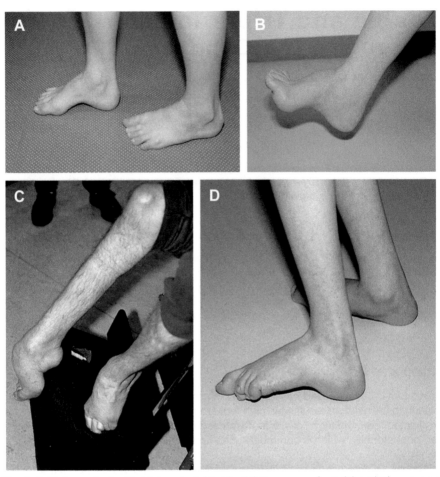

Fig. 1. A-01 Cavus foot with high arch right side. (*A*) Pure cavus foot; (*B*) typical cavovarus foot; (*C*) severe equinocavovarus foot; (*D*) calcaneocavus foot.

to consider the cause for an understanding of the deformity. In general, cavus foot is attributed to muscular imbalance. However, the underlying deforming mechanisms are not fully understood; especially in neurogenic cavus foot, controversial reports exist.[1,2]

Pure Cavus

Pure cavus may develop as an idiopathic or neurogenic disorder. The pathogenesis of idiopathic pure cavus foot is controversial. Some investigators suggest that fiber hypertrophy in the peroneus muscle relative to the anterior tibial muscle may lead or contribute to the increased plantar flexion of the forefoot and development of cavus deformity.[1,2] However, it is unclear why patients with idiopathic cavus foot often present fiber hypertrophy of peroneus longus muscle. Another possible explanation for the development of cavus foot is that peroneal longus muscle as a plantar flexor is used for the compensation of weak plantar flexor muscles (gastrocsoleus, toe flexors) leading to muscular imbalance and increased plantar flexion of the forefoot (cavus).

Table 1
Types of cavus deformities

Cavus Deformity	Cause	Pathogenesis	Clinical Findings	Radiographic Findings
"Pure" cavus	• Idiopathic • Neurogenic (rare)	• Unknown • Isolated hypertrophy of peroneus longus muscle • Neurogenic (muscular imbalance, weakness of dorsiflexors, and peroneus brevis)	Increased arch without concomitant deformity	Increased arch
Cavovarus	• Neurogenic CMT, CP, hereditary spastic paraplegia, dystrophia myotonica, spinal muscular atrophy • Idiopathic	Muscular imbalance, weakness of dorsiflexors and peroneus brevis	(Hindfoot equinus) Drop foot Hindfoot varus Cavus Forefoot pronation Claw toes	"Shortened calcaneus" open sinus tarsi "Double dome" sign Dorsal rotation of fibula High-arch plantar flexed first ray Claw toes
Equinocavovarus	• Congenital, residual • Neurogenic Athrogryposis, spina bifida, CP, traumatic brain injury, apoplexy, dystrophia myotonica, hereditary spastic paraplegia, tethered cord, diastematomyelia, paraplegia • Posttraumatic (eg, compartment syndrome)	• Unknown (congenital) • Muscular imbalance (neurogenic) overactivity of plantar flexors, tibialis posterior muscle	Hindfoot equinus Hindfoot varus Cavus adductus Forefoot supination	"Shortened calcaneus" open sinus tarsi "Double dome" sign Dorsal rotation of fibula Hindfoot equinus High-arch plantar flexed first ray Claw toes
Calcaneocavus	Neurogenic Iatrogenic • Iatrogenic (eg, after tendoachilles lengthening) • Neurogenic (eg, MMC, tethered cord, CP)	• Muscular imbalance (weakness of calf muscles, overactivity of dorsiflexors, toe flexor plantar flexion substitution) • Weakness of the calf muscles after overlengthening	Cavus Hindfoot dorsiflexed (additional varus or valgus deformity of the hindfoot) (additional deformity of the forefoot)	Increased calcaneal pitch Hindfoot varus/valgus High arch

Abbreviations: CMT, Charcot-Marie-Tooth; CP, cerebral palsy; MMC, myelomeningocele.

Cavovarus

Pathogenesis of cavovarus foot is complex and also not fully understood. Different hypotheses exist in the literature.[3–5] Because cavovarus foot deformity is most commonly found in patients with Charcot-Marie-Tooth (CMT),[6] this section is focused on the pathogenesis of cavovarus foot in CMT and related syndromes.

The most popular theory is the imbalance between the peroneus longus muscle and the weak anterior tibialis muscle couple accompanied by an imbalance between posterior tibial muscle and peroneus brevis, which shows early weakness, and strong tibialis posterior and weak peroneus brevis couple.[3] In an MRI study, Tynan and colleagues[1] found the ratio of the cross-sectional area of the peroneus longus muscle in patients with CMT and cavovarus foot to be twice of that of healthy individuals. Furthermore, the anterior tibial muscle showed more severe damage than the peroneus longus and neurogenic fiber atrophy in tibialis anterior muscle was accompanied by fiber hypertrophy in the peroneus longus muscle.[2] These findings indicate a relative imbalance between the peroneus longus muscle and the tibialis anterior muscle.[2] This discrepancy is present in most patients with CMT disease and cavovarus foot deformity. The weakness of anterior tibial muscle results in increased plantar flexion of the first ray (**Fig. 2**A) and therefore forefoot pronation and cavus. Forefoot pronation leads to hindfoot inversion due to the Cardan coupling mechanism of the foot (**Fig. 2**B). This hindfoot inversion is augmented by the muscular imbalance between the posterior tibial and the peroneus brevis muscle, which is frequently involved in early degeneration. The peroneus longus muscle tries to support the peroneus brevis in eversion of the hindfoot, which leads to further plantar flexion of the first ray. Because of a weak anterior tibial tendon that leads to drop foot, the long toe extensors try to compensate for this deficiency, which causes the clinically often seen so-called extensor substitution (**Fig. 2**C). This extensor substitution leads to hyperextension in the metatarsophalangeal joints, and the long toe flexors pull the end phalanges into plantar flexion. In combination with the concomitant loss of activity of the intrinsic foot muscles this leads to claw toes.

Equinocavovarus

Neurogenic equinocavovarus may be seen in various neurological disorders, especially in patients with cerebral palsy, hereditary spastic paraplegia, stroke, or postcompartment syndrome. Again, muscular imbalance plays a central role in the development of this foot deformity. Spasticity or overactivity of the calf muscles lead to equinus of the hindfoot. Hindfoot varus is commonly caused by overactivity of the posterior tibial tendon. The peroneus brevis muscle is not able to compensate

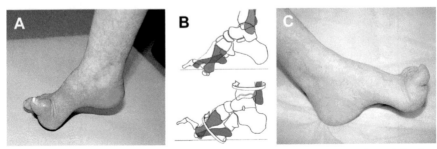

Fig. 2. (*A*) Plantar flexion of the first ray and claw toe; (*B*) the Cardan coupling of the foot; (*C*) extensor substitution.

this overactivity. Owing to overactivity of the calf muscles, there is a relative weakness of dorsiflexors, especially the anterior tibial muscle, in many patients with neurogenic equinocavovarus, leading to plantar flexion of the forefoot and cavus deformity; this is augmented by the peroneus longus muscle that is trying to help the peroneus brevis tendon to evert the hindfoot but causes further plantar flexion of the first metatarsal and therefore increase of cavus. Other patients present with combined anterior and posterior tibial muscle spasticity, which leads to hindfoot inversion and forefoot supination.

Calcaneocavus

Calcaneocavus is mostly caused by muscular imbalance between the dorsiflexors and the calf muscles. In most of the cases weakness of the triceps surae (palsy, atrophy, or overlength [iatrogenic]) is the underlying pathologic condition. Uncommonly overactivity or spasticity of the anterior tibial muscle may lead to calcaneal gait, especially in combination with weakness of the calf muscles. To enlarge the foot contact area on the ground and to compensate plantar flexor deficiency, the long toe flexors are usually activated abnormally (flexor substitution); this leads to plantar flexion of the forefoot and the development of cavus. These sagittal plane findings may be accompanied by various other deformities such as hindfoot valgus or varus and forefoot adduction or abduction depending on the underlying pathologic condition.

TREATMENT STRATEGIES
General Treatment Considerations

The aim of surgical correction should be the restoration of normal function and creation of a plantigrade foot. Bony and soft tissue procedures may be used for the correction of cavus foot deformity. Commonly there is need for combined soft tissue and bony surgery to achieve adequate correction. In general, cavus foot deformity correction consists of 2 main components: correction of the structural deformity and balancing.[4,7–10] Present deformity should be corrected by release or lengthening of soft tissue structures, or in case of bony deformity, by osteotomy or arthrodesis.[4,7–10] However, cavus deformity tends to recur if the underlying pathologic condition is not eliminated using balancing procedures (tendon transfers).[11] Tendon transfers may be used as active transfers to restore active joint function or as balancing tenodesis in cases in which restoration is not possible.[7]

The authors suggest the following general approach for correction of cavus foot:

1. Prepare all tendon transfers
2. Perform release or lengthening surgery for deformity correction
3. Correct hindfoot (osteotomy or arthrodesis)
4. Correct forefoot (osteotomy or arthrodesis)
5. Fix tendon transfers

To achieve optimal treatment results, extensive and thorough preoperative planning consisting of clinical and radiographic examinations as well as functional and dynamic testing (dynamic pedobarography[12] and 3-dimensional foot and gait analysis[13]) is essential.[4,10,11]

Specific Treatment Considerations

Pure cavus
Pure cavus should only be corrected when it is symptomatic (pain, swing phase clearance problems). Surgical treatment of symptomatic pure cavus seems to be relatively easy because correction is done in the sagittal plane only. However, different potential

Table 2
Treatment strategy for surgical management of cavovarus foot

Components of Cavovarus Foot Deformity	Surgical Strategy	Procedures
Weakness of TA and PB	Support TA and PB	Posterior tendon transfers
Hindfoot varus	Correct hindfoot varus	Chopart, triple, Lambrinudi arthrodesis Dwyer osteotomy
High arch	Reduce high arch and increase foot length	(Plantar fascia release) Chopart arthrodesis Cole osteotomy
Plantar flexed first metatarsal	Redorsiflex first metatarsal	Jones procedure, extension osteotomy of the first metatarsal
Claw toes	Correct claw toes	Jones procedure, tenotomy of long toe flexors, Hibbs procedure
Extensor substitution	Improve active dorsiflexion	T-SPOTT, POTT

Abbreviations: PB, peroneus brevis; POTT, posterior tibial tendon transfer; TA, tibialis anterior; T-SPOTT, total split posterior tibial tendon transfer.

sources for failure of treatment exist. It is controversial whether a plantar fascia release should be performed before any bony correction is done. The authors frequently perform the plantar fascia release before adding bony correction. In patients with mild involvement, especially children, this procedure may lead to correction of cavus deformity. In most of the patients this procedure does not lead to adequate correction. Therefore, additional bony correction is done. The following procedures have the potential to correct cavus deformity:

- Extension osteotomy first ray (only if there is isolated involvement of the first metatarsal)[14]
- Cole osteotomy[15]
- Chopart arthrodesis (± dorsal-based wedge)

Cavovarus foot
For the treatment of cavovarus foot the authors suggest a standardized protocol including a combination of soft tissue and bony procedures. **Table 2** summarizes the treatment strategy for surgical correction of cavovarus foot deformity.

For the treatment of weak anterior tibial muscle and peroneus brevis muscle, the authors suggest the T-SPOTT (total split posterior tibial tendon transfer) procedure, which was formerly published.[4,7,9] The complete posterior tibial tendon is released, split into 2 halves, transferred through the interosseous membrane anteriorly, and fixed to the anterior tibial tendon and the peroneus brevis tendon; this leads to elimination of the influence of tibialis posterior muscle on hindfoot varus and augmentation of dorsiflexion. The authors consider preparing the tendon transfers before performing hindfoot and forefoot correction and to fix the transfers at the end of the surgery.

The correction of hindfoot varus plays a central role in the correction of cavovarus foot deformity, and it can be achieved by using osteotomies (joint sparing) or arthrodesis. Regardless the strategy chosen, it is essential to restore normal hindfoot anatomy and congruence of ankle joint. The authors frequently perform Chopart arthrodesis rather than Dwyer[16] osteotomy due to different reasons. First, complete correction of the hindfoot deformity is difficult to achieve by Dwyer osteotomy[16] because multiplanar deformity is present and Dwyer osteotomy only corrects the varus component. Furthermore, sparing the Chopart joint may lead to recurrence of deformity or collapse into planovalgus foot, especially because posterior tibial muscle is eliminated completely. In severe deformities, triple arthrodesis may be needed to achieve acceptable correction.[17–19] In patients showing ventral impingement at the ankle with limited dorsiflexion or severe hindfoot equinus a modified Lambrinudi procedure is carried out for correction.[20] Concerning cavus component, there is controversy if soft tissue procedures (eg, plantar fascia release[21]) for the correction of cavus component should be carried out. On one hand, complete correction is rarely achieved by soft tissue procedures; on the other hand, collapse of the foot arch due to elimination of arch stabilization mechanisms should be discussed. However, plantar fascia release may reduce deformity and therefore the amount of bony correction. The authors routinely perform Steindler plantar fascia release in most of the patients with cavovarus deformity.[21] Bony procedures for the correction of cavus component include Cole osteotomy[15] or Chopart arthrodesis. In cases of isolated plantar flexed first metatarsal, extension osteotomy of the first metatarsal[14] is rather considered for correction. The next step is the correction of the first ray by modified Jones procedure,[22,23] which eliminates the overactivity of extensor hallucis longus muscle and corrects the claw toe deformity of the first toe. In cases with persistent plantar flexion of the first metatarsal, extension osteotomy is performed.[14] Afterward, gastrocsoleus length should be evaluated. Rare cases show additional shortening of the calf muscles, which may need aponeurotic calf muscle lengthening or Achilles tendon lengthening. Furthermore, rotation deformities of the tibia should be identified and corrected by supramalleolar osteotomy at this time. Afterward claw toes are corrected by tenotomy of the toe flexors, proximal interphalangeal (PIP) fusions, or Hibbs procedure.[24] In the end the tendon transfers are fixed while the foot is held in corrected position.

Equinocavovarus foot

Treatment of neurogenic and congenital equinocavovarus deformity is based on a combined soft tissue and bony approach. Although tendon transfers are carried out in combination with osteotomies or fusions in neurogenic equinocavovarus, tendon transfer surgery is of minor importance for the correction of recurrent congenital clubfoot, where release surgery is combined with bony procedures. It is essential to evaluate the mechanism of the pathologic condition and therefore the underlying cause for the correction of neurogenic equinocavovarus.

Analogous to what was considered for the treatment of cavovarus deformity, the cavovarus component may be corrected by osteotomies or fusions in the hindfoot and midfoot. Cavus component is corrected by Cole osteotomy,[15] Chopart arthrodesis, or in cases with isolated involvement of the first metatarsal ray by extension osteotomy of the first metatarsal.[14] Before the correction, a plantar fascia release may be carried out. Hindfoot varus may be corrected during Chopart arthrodesis, whereas Cole osteotomy for cavus correction does not influence hindfoot position and a Dwyer osteotomy must be added to achieve correction of the hindfoot. In more severe cases, triple[17–19] or Lambrinudi arthrodesis[20] is needed for complete correction.

There is a significant difference between the balancing strategy of cavovarus foot and equinocavovarus foot when considering the underlying pathologic condition.[7] In contrast to muscular imbalance, which is caused by atrophy, transfer of complete tendons in spastic deformities should not be carried out due to the danger for overcorrection. Because cavus and varus components are results of overactivity of the tibialis posterior muscle ± long toe flexors, balancing should include posterior tibial muscle using SPOTT (split posterior tibial tendon transfer) to the lateral border of the foot,[25,26] either through the interosseous membrane (in cases showing concomitant drop foot) or by circumtibial transfer.[27] The hindfoot varus during stance phase is sometimes accompanied by forefoot supination during swing phase. In those cases, additional split anterior tibial tendon transfer to the peroneus tertius or the cuboid bone is considered.[7,28–30]

Equinus of the hindfoot should be corrected by intramuscular aponeurotic gastrocsoleus lengthening in mildly involved cases.[31] More severe cases with isolated gastrocnemius involvement may be corrected by gastrocnemius recession (Strayer procedure).[32] Fixed severe equinus should be treated by Achilles tendon lengthening.[28] In cases in which plantigrade position of the ankle is not possible by soft tissue procedures or in cases with ventral impingement in the ankle, the authors suggest Lambrinudi arthrodesis.[20] In cases with severe drop foot transfer of the long toe flexors to the dorsum of the foot may be additionally carried out.[33–35] **Table 3** summarizes the treatment strategies for the correction of equinocavovarus foot deformity.

Calcaneocavus foot

The surgical treatment of paralytic or iatrogenic calcaneocavus foot is a challenge, and various controversial strategies for its treatment exist in the literature. The weakness or overlength of the calf muscles represents the central problem in calcaneocavus foot. Therefore, the most important treatment goal is the augmentation of Achilles tendon by tendon transfers. Georgiadis and Aronson[36] described a method for the transfer

Table 3
Treatment strategy for surgical management of equinocavovarus foot

Components of Equinocavovarus Foot Deformity	Surgical Strategy	Procedures
Overactivity of tibialis posterior	Reduce TP medially, support PB laterally	Posterior tibial tendon transfers
Hindfoot varus	Correct hindfoot varus	Chopart, triple, Lambrinudi arthrodesis Dwyer osteotomy
High arch	Reduce high arch and increase foot length	(Plantar fascia release) Chopart arthrodesis Cole osteotomy
Equinus	Correct equinus	Aponeurotic gastrocsoleus recession Gastrocnemius recession (Strayer) Achilles tendon lengthening Lambrinudi arthrodesis
Drop foot	Improve active dorsiflexion	Hiroshima procedure, modified SPOTT (transmembrane)
Claw toes	Correct claw toes	Jones procedure, tenotomy of long toe flexors, Hibbs procedure

Abbreviations: PB, peroneus brevis; TP, tibialis posterior.

of complete anterior tibial tendon to the calcaneus to strengthen the calf muscles in patients with spina bifida and calcaneal gait. Park and colleagues[37] reported satisfactory results after anterior tibial tendon transfer to the Achilles tendon using 3-dimensional gait analysis. However, Stott and colleagues[38] could show that the isolated transfer of the anterior tibial tendon could not prevent the excessive ankle dorsiflexion during stance phase and that additional pretibial ankle-foot orthosis was necessary to achieve optimum gait function. More encouraging results were reported by DiCesare and colleagues,[39] who transferred 1 to 5 tendons in patients with postpolio syndrome, but again no significant improvement in gait analysis parameters could be found. The authors consider transfer of all tendons (tibialis anterior and posterior, peroneus brevis and longus, and extensor digitorum and hallucis longus) to the Achilles tendon sparing the long toe flexors, which may be used for a secondary Hiroshima procedure in case of postoperative drop foot.[40] The transfers were done in combination with an inverse Lambrinudi-type arthrodesis for correction of concomitant other deformities. Excellent functional results were found in 6 patients, of which 2 needed secondary toe flexor transfer due to secondary drop foot.[40]

However, regardless the technique chosen, the key for surgical treatment of calcaneal foot is to provide enough plantar flexor strength. Enough tendons should be transferred, therefore. The correction of cavus deformity depends on the concomitant other hindfoot deformity (see earlier).

Surgical technique
Surgical approaches and technique are described for cavovarus foot deformity in CMT. First, the posterior tibial tendon is exposed at its insertion at the navicular bone (**Fig. 3**A) and released. At the medial shank, the tendon is pulled out through another incision (**Fig. 3**B); it can be found lying under the flexor digitorum longus tendon directly behind the tibia. The tendon is afterward split into 2 halves (**Fig. 3**C), which are tagged and transferred through the interosseous membrane into the extensor compartment (**Fig. 3**D, E). Through a small incision anteriorly over the extensor compartment, the tendons can be pulled out (**Fig. 3**F). Back to the approach at the medial aspect of the foot, the anterior tibial tendon is identified (**Fig. 3**G). Through another incision over the origin of the plantar fascia at the calcaneus, the plantar fascia release according to Steindler[21] is carried out. At the lateral border of the foot another incision is performed. The incision may be slightly s-shaped, starts about 1 cm distally from the malleolus lateralis, and leads to the dorsum of the foot. After identification of the sural nerve, the tendon sheaths of the peroneal tendons are incised. The peroneus longus tendon is identified by dorsiflexion and plantar flexion of the first metatarsal and tenotomized or lengthened, whereas the peroneus brevis tendon is tagged. Back to medial aspect of the foot, one-half of the posterior tibial tendon is transferred distally beneath the retinaculum through the tendon sheath of the anterior tibial tendon (**Fig. 3**H). At the lateral aspect of the foot, the sheath of the long toe extensors is incised, and the other tendon half of tibialis posterior is transferred to the lateral border of the foot beneath the retinaculum through the sheath of toe extensor tendons (**Fig. 3**I, J). Fixation of transfers is done at the end of the surgery.

After preparation of tendon transfers, correction of the hindfoot and midfoot deformity follows. The authors prefer Chopart arthrodesis in most of the cases because it allows 3-dimensional correction. Capsule of Chopart joint is opened medially and laterally, and cartilage from the talonavicular as well as the calcaneocuboid joint is removed with a shaped chisel (**Fig. 3**K–O). In general, reorientation and fusion after release and removal of cartilage leads to sufficient correction in all 3 planes. In cases

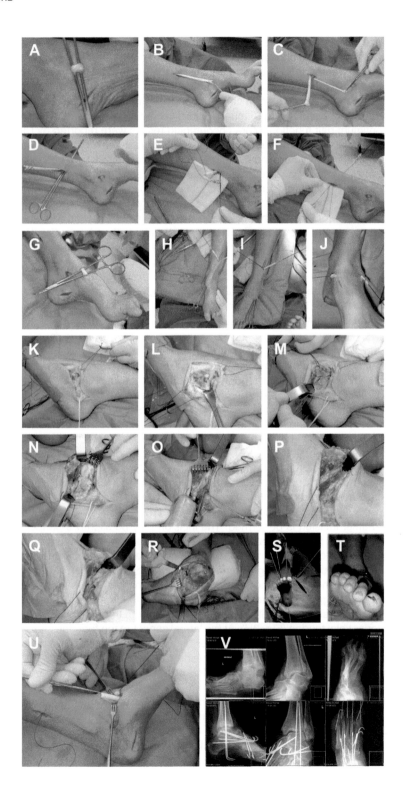

showing severe cavus deformity, an additional dorsal-based wedge may be taken to achieve complete correction (**Fig. 3**P, Q). If complete correction of hindfoot varus is not possible by Chopart fusion or in case of severe instability in the subtalar, joint triple arthrodesis[17–19] may be needed and a lateral-based wedge can be resected from the subtalar joint in severe hindfoot varus, possibly through the same lateral approach (**Fig. 3**R). In cases in which the talus impinges at the tibia or bony fixed hindfoot equinus Lambrinudi arthrodesis[20] is added taking a ventral-based wedge from the subtalar joint with an oscillating bone saw or chisel. Afterward the hindfoot is reorientated in corrected position. During this step it is of importance not to try to correct plantar flexed position of the first metatarsal. The authors consider neutral position or slight eversion of the heel, whereas the forefoot and midfoot are held in pronation and neutral position concerning forefoot abduction and adduction. K-wire fixation is first done at the calcaneocuboid joint with 2 K-wires (2.5 mm for adults, 2.2 mm for children and adolescents). Afterward the talonavicular joint is fixed with 2 more K-wires, and in cases with triple or Lambrinudi arthrodesis 2 additional wires are used to fix the calcaneus to the talus (**Fig. 3**S). Radiographs are done to check the correction and the position of K-wires. A hindfoot correction in all 3 planes should be achieved, but in most of the cases plantar flexed first ray remains (**Fig. 3**T). A Silfverskiöld test is then performed to detect any calf muscle shortness. In mild cases an intramuscular gastroc(soleus) recession is preferred (Baumann[28] and Strayer[29] procedures), whereas in rare severe cases Achilles tendon lengthening may be needed to achieve correction.

The next step of the surgery is the correction of the first ray. In cases showing dynamic claw first claw toe with hyperextension in the first metatarsophalangeal joint,[14] the authors consider performing the modified Jones procedure,[22,23] which includes the transfer of the extensor hallucis longus to the first metatarsal bone and a fusion of the first interphalangeal joint. For the correction of plantar flexion of the first metatarsal extension osteotomy of the first metatarsal is done.[14] The osteotomy is closed and fixed with an angle stable locking plate or with 1 or 2 crossing K-wires.

Afterward the tendon transfers are sutured. Laterally one-half of the posterior tibial tendon is sutured to the peroneus brevis tendon. At the medial aspect of the foot the other half of the tendon is sutured to the anterior tibial tendon in the same technique (**Fig. 3**U). Claw toes may then be corrected with tenotomy of the flexor tendons and/or PIP fusions. At the end of the surgery, tibial torsion and foot alignment should be checked. Very rare cases may present abnormal tibial torsion needing supramalleolar derotation osteotomy. Final radiographs are obtained (**Fig. 3**V).

Fig. 3. (A) Posterior tibial tendon; (B) pulled out posterior tibial tendon; (C) tendon is split in 2 halves; (D) a long slim forcep is placed through the intraosseous membrane; (E) the threads are pulled through the intraosseous membrane; (F) the tendons are pulled through; (G) anterior tibial tendon; (H) medial tendon half runs with the anterior tibial tendon under the retinaculum; (I) lateral tendon half runs with the extensor digitorum under the retinaculum; (J) correct tendon position after the rerouting; (K) lateral approach with the sural nerve in the loop; (L) extensor digitorum brevis release; (M) the calcaneocuboid joint; (N) retractors give good exposure of the lateral Chopart joint; (O) removal of the joint surfaces using an oscillating saw; (P) joints are removed; (Q) arthrodesis with good alignment; (R) if needed the approach gives good exposure of the subtalar also; (S) typical situation after placing the K-wires; (T) lateral tendon-to-tendon fixation; (T) after fixing the hindfoot in corrected position the first ray is even more plantarized; (U) elongated anterior tibial tendon pulled out for augmentation with the medial tendon half; (V) position of the wires in a sophisticated case of CMT.

OUTCOME
Cavovarus

A 42-year-old patient with CMT is presented. He suffered from bilateral severe cavovarus foot with the left side more involved (**Fig. 4**A, B) without the ability to walk without custom-made shoes. He underwent surgery on the left side including Steindler procedure,[21] modified Jones procedure,[22,23] T-SPOTT, a Chopart fusion, and an extension osteotomy of the first metatarsal[14] and tenotomies for correction of DII-DV (**Fig. 4**C). **Fig. 4**D and E shows the 1-year postoperative outcome, where a good clinical, functional, and radiographic result could be found. The patient also came for the treatment of the right side.

Equinocavovarus

A 32-year-old patient with polio is presented. He suffered from unilateral severe equinocavovarus foot on the left side (**Fig. 4**F–H) and could not walk without custom-made shoes. He underwent massive acute correction including Steindler procedure,[21]

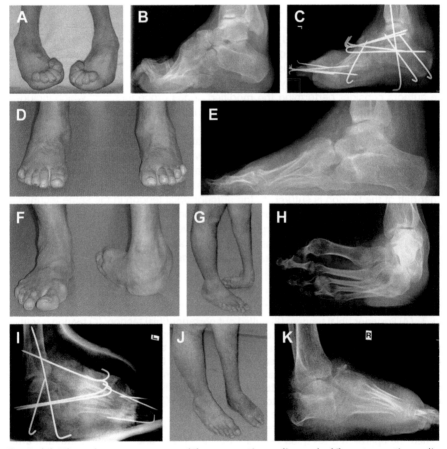

Fig. 4. (A) Bilateral severe cavovarus; (B) preoperative radiograph; (C) postoperative radiograph; (D) postoperative result after correction; (E) radiograph after treatment; (F) severe polio cavovarus; (G) lateral aspect; (H) preoperative radiograph; (I) postoperative radiograph; (J) postoperative result after correction; (K) radiograph after treatment.

modified Jones procedure,[22,23] T-SPOTT, a triple fusion, and an extension osteotomy of the first metatarsal[14] and tenotomies for correction of DII-DV (**Fig. 4I**). **Fig. 4**J and K shows the 1-year postoperative outcome, where a good clinical, functional, and radiographic result could be found.

SUMMARY

The surgical treatment of cavus foot is a challenge. The cavus foot is frequently accompanied by different other components of foot deformity and only rarely seen in its pure form. The most common types of cavus foot are the pure cavus, the cavovarus, the equinocavovarus, and the calcaneocavus foot. For a successful surgical treatment of these cavus-type deformities, a detailed evaluation of the pathomechanics of the deformity and its underlying cause is essential. Treatment strategy considers pathomechanics and aims to create a plantigrade and well-balanced foot. Bony procedures (osteotomies and/or fusions) and soft tissue procedures (tendon/muscle lengthenings or releases) for the correction of the deformity are routinely combined with tendon transfers for the elimination of the underlying pathologic condition and for balancing in neurogenic cavus foot. Although pure cavus represents a deformity that includes only 1 plane, cavovarus, equinocavovarus, and calcaneocavus commonly present with multiplanar deformities, which needs a complex reconstruction. Treatment strategies for the successful correction of all 4 types of cavus foot according to the underlying pathologic condition are presented and discussed in detail in this investigation.

CLINICS CARE POINTS

- If using K-wires for osteosynthesis a custom-made cast should be made and changed every 2 weeks.
- A period of 6 weeks without weight-bearing is recommended.
- The authors recommend a 4-step surgical procedure,
  1. Prepare tendon transfers
  2. Correct hindfoot
  3. Correct first metatarsal
  4. Fix all tendon transfers

DISCLAIMER

The author has nothing to disclose.

REFERENCES

1. Tynan MC, Klenerman L, Helliwell TR, et al. Investigation of muscle imbalance in the leg in symptomatic forefoot pes cavus: a multidisciplinary study. Foot Ankle 1992;13:489–501.
2. Helliwell TR, Tynan M, Hayward M, et al. The pathology of the lower leg muscles in pure forefoot pes cavus. Acta Neuropathol 1995;89(6):552–9.
3. Mann RA, Missirian J. Pathophysiology of charcot-marie-tooth disease. Clin Orthop Relat Res 1988;234:221–8.

4. Wenz W, Dreher T. Charcot-marie-tooth disease and the cavovarus foot. In: Pinzur MS, editor. Orthopaedic knowledge update – foot and ankle. AAOS; 2008. p. 291–306.
5. Azmaipairashvili Z, Riddle EC, Scavina M, et al. Correction of cavovarus foot deformity in Charcot-Marie-Tooth disease. J Pediatr Orthop 2005;25:360–5.
6. Nagai MK, Chan G, Guille JT, et al. Prevalence of Charcot-Marie-Tooth Disease in patients who have bilateral cavovarus feet. J Pediatr Orthop 2006;26:438–43.
7. Dreher T, Wenz W. Tendon transfers for the balancing of hind and mid-foot deformities in adults and children. Tech Foot Ankle Surg 2009;8:178–89.
8. Ward CM, Dolan LA, Bennett DL, et al. Long-term results of reconstruction for treatment of a flexible cavovarus foot in Charcot-Marie-Tooth disease. J Bone Joint Surg Am 2008;90:2631–42.
9. Dreher T, Hagmann S, Wenz W. Reconstruction of multiplanar deformity of the hind- and midfoot with internal fixation techniques. Foot Ankle Clin 2009;14: 489–531.
10. Leeuwesteijn AE, de Visser E, Louwerens JW. Flexible cavovarus feet in Charcot-Marie-Tooth disease treated with first ray proximal dorsiflexion osteotomy combined with soft tissue surgery: a short-term to mid-term outcome study. Foot Ankle Surg 2010;16:142–7.
11. Jahss MH. Evaluation of the cavus foot for orthopedic treatment. Clin Orthop Rel Res 1983;181:52–63.
12. Metaxiotis D, Accles W, Pappas A, et al. Dynamic pedobarography (DPB) in operative management of cavovarus foot deformity. Foot Ankle Int 2000;21: 935–47.
13. Simon J, Doederlein L, McIntosh AS, et al. The Heidelberg foot measurement method: development, description and assessment. Gait Posture 2006;23: 411–24.
14. Tubby AH. Deformities including diseases of bones and joints. ed 2. London, England: MacMillan; 1912.
15. Cole WH. The treatment of claw foot. J Bone Joint Surg 1940;22:895–908.
16. Dwyer FC. The present status of the problem of pes cavus. Clin Orthop Relat Res 1975;106:254–75.
17. Hoke M. An operation for stabilizing paralytic feet. J Orthop Surg (Hong Kong) 1921;3:494.
18. Wetmore RS, Drennan JC. Long-term results of triple arthrodesis in Charcot-Marie-Tooth disease. J Bone Joint Surg Am 1989;71:417–22.
19. Vlachou M, Dimitriadis D. Results of triple arthrodesis in children and adolescents. Acta Orthop Belg 2009;75:380–8.
20. Lambrinudi C. New operation for drop foot. Br J Surg 1927;15:193.
21. Steindler A. The treatment of pes cavus (hollow claw foot). Arch Surg 1921;2: 325–37.
22. Jones R. An Operation for Paralytic Calcaneo-Cavus. Am J Orthop Surg 1908; 190:371–6.
23. DePalma L, Colonna E, Travasi M. The modified Jones procedure for pes cavovarus with claw hallux. J Foot Ankle Surg 1997;36:279–83.
24. Hibbs RA. An operation for claw foot. J Am Med Assoc 1919;73:1583–5.
25. O'Byrne JM, Kennedy A, Jenkinson A, et al. Split tibialis posterior tendon transfer in the treatment of spastic equinovarus foot. J Pediatr Orthop 1997;17:481–5.
26. Mulier T, Moens P, Molenaers G, et al. Split posterior tibial tendon transfer through the interosseus membrane in spastic equinovarus deformity. Foot Ankle Int 1995; 16:754–9.

27. Qian JG, Yao WH, Qian CZ. A long-term follow-up result of posterior tibialis muscle transfer for foot-drop in leprosy patients. Zhongguo Xiu Fu Chong Jian Wai Ke Za Zhi 2003;17:240–1.
28. Edwards P, Hsu J. SPLATT combined with tendo achilles lengthening for spastic equinovarus in adults: results and predictors of surgical outcome. Foot Ankle 1993;14:335–8.
29. Hoffer MM, Reiswig JA, Garrett AM, et al. The split anterior tibial tendon transfer in the treatment of spastic varus hindfoot of childhood. Orthop Clin North Am 1974; 5:31–8.
30. Vogt JC. Split anterior tibial transfer for spastic equinovarus foot deformity: retrospective study of 73 operated feet. J Foot Ankle Surg 1998;37:2–7.
31. Baumann JU, Koch HG: Ventrale aponeurotische Verlängerung des Musculus gastrocnemius Operative Orthopädie und Traumatologie 1989;4:254-258.
32. Strayer LM. Gastrocnemius recession: a five-year report of cases. J Bone Joint Surg Am 1958;40:1019–30.
33. Ono K, Hiroshima K, Tada K, et al. Anterior transfer of the toe flexors for equinovarus deformity of the foot. Int Orthop 1980;4:225–9.
34. Hiroshima K, Hamada S, Shimizu N, et al. Anterior transfer of the long toe flexors for the treatment of spastic equinovarus and equinus foot in cerebral palsy. J Pediatr Orthop 1988;8:164–8.
35. Morita S, Yamamoto H, Furuya K. Anterior transfer of the toe flexors for equinovarus deformity due to hemiplegia. J Bone Joint Surg Br 1994;76:447–9.
36. Georgiadis GM, Aronson DD. Posterior transfer of the anterior tibial tendon in children who have a myelomeningocele. J Bone Joint Surg Am 1990;72:792.
37. Park KB, Park HW, Joo SY, et al. Surgical treatment of calcaneal deformity in a select group of patients with myelomeningocele. J Bone Joint Surg Am 2008; 90:2149–59.
38. Stott NS, Zionts LE, Gronley JK, et al. Tibialis anterior transfer for calcaneal deformity: a postoperative gait analysis. J Pediatr Orthop 1996;16:792–8.
39. DiCesare PE, Young S, Perry J, et al. Perimalleolar tendon transfer to the os calcis for triceps surae insufficiency in patients with postpolio syndrome. Clin Orthop Relat Res 1995;310:111–9.
40. Wenz W, Bruckner T, Akbar M. Complete tendon transfer and inverse Lambrinudi arthrodesis: preliminary results of a new technique for the treatment of paralytic pes calcaneus. Foot Ankle Int 2008;29:683–9.

Arthrodesis in the Deformed Charcot Foot

Dov Lagus Rosemberg, MD[a,b,c,d],*, Rafael Barban Sposeto, MS, MD[a],
Alexandre Leme Godoy-Santos, PhD, MD[a,b]

KEYWORDS

- Charcot foot • Deformity • Dislocation • Arthrodesis • Bone graft

KEY POINTS

- Despite the midfoot being the most affected region of the foot and ankle, the hindfoot (34%) and the ankle (11%) also show a high incidence of neuroarthopathy.
- Tibiotalocalcaneal arthrodesis with nails or a double plate is a good strategy for correcting and treating deformities in the ankle and hindfoot of Charcot neuroarthropathy.
- When the defect is considered too big to use a tricortical structured autograft, a femoral head graft can be used.
- The loss of a segment of bone, such as the talus, is a critical condition, and arthrodesis is a tool to attempt to maintain the foot in a plantigrade, stable, and functional position, sometimes despite causing limb shortening.

INTRODUCTION

Charcot's neuroarthropathy (CN) is a noninfective, destructive process occurring in patients with an inability to sense pain because of peripheral neuropathy with a devastating impact on a patient's mobility and quality of life. The physiopathology begins with intense swelling, associated with fractures and progressive dislocations, mainly in the foot and ankle. At the end of the inflammatory phase, bone healing occurs, and the residual deformity is established. Currently, diabetes mellitus (DM) is the most important cause.

The American Diabetes Association estimated that nearly 7.8% of the population of the United States is affected by DM, with CN affecting around 8.5 per 1000 of the

[a] Departamento de Ortopedia e Traumatologia, Hospital das Clínicas, Faculdade de Medicina, Universidade de São Paulo, São Paulo, Dr. Ovídio Pires de Campos, 333 - Cerqueira César, São Paulo, São Paulo 05403-010, Brazil; [b] Hospital Israelita Albert Einstein, São Paulo, Av. Albert Einstein, 627/701 - Morumbi, São Paulo - SP, 05652-900, Brazil; [c] International Scholar at the Midwest Orthopedics at Rush (MOR), 1620 W. Harrison St., Chicago, IL, 6012, USA; [d] RUSH-IBTS International Fellowship Program, 1620 W. Harrison St., Chicago, IL, 6012, USA
* Corresponding author. R. Dr. Ovídio Pires de Campos, 333 - Cerqueira César, São Paulo, São Paulo 05403-010, Brazil.
E-mail address: dr.dovr@gmail.com

Foot Ankle Clin N Am 27 (2022) 835–846
https://doi.org/10.1016/j.fcl.2022.08.005

diabetic population per year.[1] Ulceration and infection are common; CN is associated with a rate of major amputation of 15%, which increases from 35% to 67% in patients with CN who present with an associated ulcer.[2] Despite the midfoot being the most affected region of the foot and ankle, the hindfoot (34%) and ankle (11%) also show a high incidence of pathology.[3]

Treatment of the Charcot joint is diverse and includes total contact casting, shoewear modifications, medication, and surgical correction. The primary indications for surgery are recurrent ulceration, substantial deformity, deep infection, and intractable pain. Common complications include nonunion, wound breakdown, and infection.[1] Arthrodesis is indicated in severe Charcot joint deformity with significant skeletal instability. Internal fixation is more popular than external fixation in the absence of osteomyelitis, significant bone defect, poor bone quality, and poor soft tissue coverage. Various methods of internal fixation have been evaluated, including retrograde intramedullary nails, screws, and plates.[4]

MANAGING THE HINDFOOT CHARCOT

The CN is a severe pathology leading to fractures, subluxations and dislocations, and ankle and foot architecture modifications with deformities, most affecting weight distribution.[5] In these situations, every step during gait becomes a trauma to the foot, affecting the segment's bone and soft tissues, potentially ending up in lesions associated with ulcers and infection.[6]

Patients with ulcers and deformities related to CN have impaired mobility and quality of life, with a high chance of amputation.[7,8] Patients with DM, ulcer, infection, and CN have a rate of up to 67% of amputation in this scenario, and most of the investigators consider them high-risk limb salvage patients.[4,5,9] Therefore, when the patient has already developed a deformity that is be braceable, the treatment strategy will aim at the correction of the foot and ankle positions, providing a stable and plantigrade foot with better weight-bearing distribution, less chance of ulceration, lesions, and amputations.[9–11] Most cases have severe joint deformities with irreversible damage, and arthrodesis is the most suitable option for reconstruction.[5,8,9,12] Around 30% of the foot and ankle CN is located in the hindfoot and 10% in the ankle.[13] The correction and stabilization of tibiotalar and subtalar joints are often required in these situations, with tibiotalocalcaneal (TTC) arthrodesis, or some variation as tibiocalcaneal (TC) arthrodesis, affording a stable, plantigrade, braceable, safer load pattern and better quality of life for these patients.[7,9,12] (**Fig. 1**). These procedures are typically done in a high-risk patient population with obesity, DM, venous and arterial vascular impairment, neuropathy (motor, sensitive, and autonomic), and cardiovascular and renal pathology thus being exposed to a high rate of complications such as malunion, nonunion, dehiscence, infection, hardware problems, and amputation.[5,9] To reach better surgical outcomes it is essential to treat these patients with a multidisciplinary approach covering all fields involved, such as endocrinologist, vascular surgeon, nephrologist, wound care specialist, physiotherapist, cardiologist, and orthopedic surgeon.[5]

Tibiotalocalcaneal Arthrodesis

Tibiotalocalcaneal arthrodesis can be fixed with screws, plates, intramedullary nails, external fixators, or with a combination of these implants.[5,14,15] Siebachmeyer and colleagues,[5] in a retrospective series of 20 patients with ankle and hindfoot CN and DM, used retrograde intramedullary nails for TTCs with excellent evolution after a mean follow-up of 25 months. All 20 patients had their members preserved, with statistical improvement in objective and subjective scores and 90% of cases showing

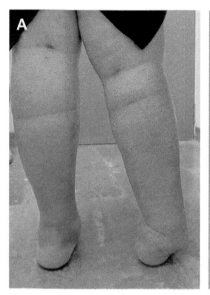
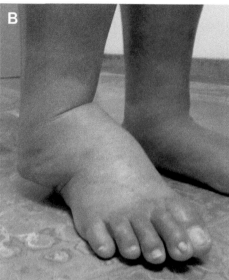

Fig. 1. Clinical presentation of an ankle CN severe deformity. This deformity is unbreaceble, with a varus ankle incompatible with a standard weight-bearing. (*A*) Posterior aspect of the right ankle, with a varus deformity, and (*B*) anterior aspect of the right ankle, with a varus deformity.

fusion. One patient could not achieve full weight-bearing during the follow-up, one nail broke and was removed, and 18% cases presented with screw migration, but there were no infections. Pinzur and colleagues[15] and Dalla and colleagues[16] showed similar outcomes. DeVries and colleagues,[17] in a retrospective study, treated 52 CN patients with TTC arthrodesis, 45 fixed with intramedullary nail, and 7 with nails combined with an external fixator. With a mean follow-up of 96 weeks, 75.6% of patients had their limbs salvaged, 48% suffered deep infection treated with debridement, and 42.3% had hardware complications. Twenty-three percent of patients ended up amputated.

These articles show some differences in outcomes, probably related to their population and fixation methods, but emphasize that TTC arthrodesis with nails is a good strategy in correcting and treating severe deformities in the ankle and hindfoot of CN.[5,18] Fixation with an intramedullary nail provides relative stability, but even better primary stability may be achieved by using nails with intrinsic compression devices or miss-a-nail compression screws. Another fixation option that provides enhanced primary stability and is in consonance with the concept of superconstructs is the use of a locking plate combined with compression screws.[10,14,19,20] There are many options to position a plate, with some plates designed to be positioned anteriorly in the ankle, others posteriorly, and others laterally.

In **Fig. 2** the authors present a patient with an Eichenholtz 3 CN of the ankle, with varus residual deformity. In this case they performed a tibiotalocalcaneal arthrodesis with a superconstruct concept using medial and lateral locked plates associated with lag screws, to enhance the stability and the chances of bone healing with the right alignment.

In **Fig. 3**, the authors present a patient with an Eichenholtz 3 CN of the ankle and hindfoot. There is a severe deformity in varus of ankle and subtalar joints and involvement of the talonavicular joint. A pantalar arthrodesis was preferred in this case due to

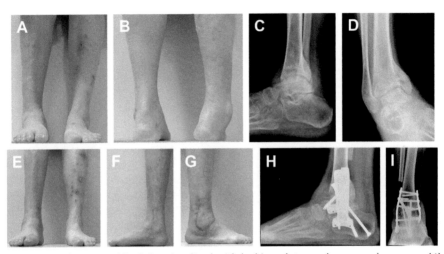

Fig. 2. CN with varus ankle deformity, fixed with locking plates and compression screw. (*A*) Anterior aspect of the right limb deformity; (*B*) posterior aspect of the right limb deformity; (*C*) lateral radiography; (*D*) AP radiography; (*E*) third month postoperative, anterior view; (*F*) third month postoperative, medial view, with adequate healing and consolidation; and (*G*) third month postoperative, lateral view, with adequate healing and consolidation; (*H*) third month postoperative, lateral radiography, with an adequate consolidation; and (*I*) third month postoperative, AP radiography, with an adequate consolidation.

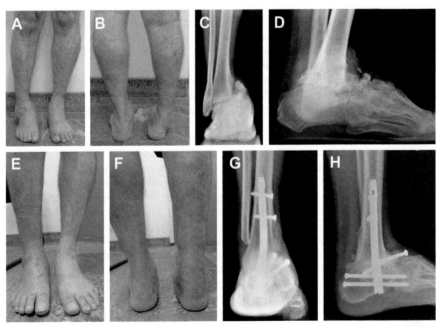

Fig. 3. TCC arthrodesis fixed with an intramedullary nail, associated with Chopart arthrodesis. (*A*) and (*B*) Clinical presentation of the ankle and hindfoot varus deformity; (*C, D*) AP and lateral radiographs showing involvement in the tibiotalar, subtalar, and talonavicular joints; (*E, F*) clinical presentation of the sixth month postoperative; (*G, H*) AP and lateral radiographs, with correction of deformity and arthrodesis consolidation.

the great power of correction in the alignment of a degenerated Chopart and to enhance overall stability.

The approach to the ankle and hindfoot in a TTC arthrodesis can be anterior, lateral (transfibular), posterior, or medial. Depending on the deformity's severity and apex, these incisions can be isolated or combined to reach the most affected segment. The most common approaches are anterior and lateral. Lateral approach allows easy access to the tibiotalar and subtalar joints.[10,14] When the patient is positioned in lateral decubitus, with the limb to be operated facing upward, the approach is developed through a single lateral incision. An osteotomy of the fibula is made above the tibiotalar joint, allowing direct visualization of the hindfoot and ankle, which are prepared and positioned. In this lateral decubitus, the surgeon has a 360° of vision of the segment, just by externally rotating the hip, allowing the control of ankle and hindfoot position. Another advantage of this positioning is that the lateral incision can be extended to the midfoot, and a medial accessory approach can be made by externally rotating the hip (**Fig. 4**).

Some severe deformities of the ankle and hindfoot impair the calcaneocuboid and talonavicular joints, and a TTC arthrodesis is insufficient to correct the deformity. In these cases, to correctly position the foot plantigrade, the surgeon needs to add these articulations into the arthrodesis (pantalar arthrodesis). If there is a medial apex deformity or prominence, a medial accessory approach might be helpful to achieve a full correction.[5,12,21]

Tibiocalcaneal Arthrodesis

In some patients with CN with loss of a significant amount of bone (usually the talus), a TTC arthrodesis cannot be accomplished. Part of these cases are related to the necrosis associated with the CN, but some others are related to severe deformity, ulcer, and talar osteomyelitis.[7,8,10,22] In the case of talar osteomyelitis, infection should be treated before a definitive stabilization with arthrodesis is attempted.[5,22] After the progress of CN stabilizes or infection is under control, correction of the ankle and hindfoot may be done, with one of the options being TC arthrodesis.[7,8,10,22] This procedure is even more challenging than TTC arthrodesis, with worst outcomes and average shortening of around 3 cm of the limb.[10]

Caravaggi and colleagues[18] presented a cohort study of 45 patients with ankle and hindfoot CN and DM. These patients were treated with a retrograde intramedullary nail for a TC arthrodesis with 5.25 years of follow-up, of them 4.44% had deep infection (that ended up in below-the-knee amputation); also 4.44% had a posttraumatic tibia fracture around the nail and a below-the-knee amputation.); 4.44% had a posttraumatic tibia fracture around the nail and a below-the-knee amputation. Twenty-two

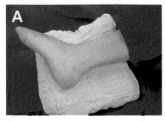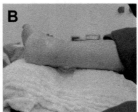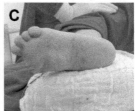

Fig. 4. Patient positioning in lateral decubitus. (*A*) Lateral view, allowing visual correction in the sagittal plane; (*B*) posterior view, allowing correction of varus/valgus; (*C*) plantar view, allowing control of adduction/abduction, supination/pronation after externally rotating the hip to reach the medial view.

percent suffered from dehiscence and superficial infection, treated with oral antibiotics. Twenty-two percent had hardware problems, and 15% needed nail removal. Eighty-six percent had their limb salvaged, with almost 95% of unions. Love and colleagues,[8] in a retrospective cohort of 18 patients with severe hindfoot and ankle disease (7 with DM and 9 with CN), showed an incidence of 44.5% of nonunions, with a higher incidence in patients with DM. Twenty-two percent of infection and 11% (2 patients) needed an amputation. Results of TC arthrodesis are worse than TCC, as shown in the articles earlier, but we should understand that the patients in situations that demand a TC arthrodesis are more critical and have the worst deformities. These outcomes are somehow expected.

Surgical approach of TC arthrodesis is similar to that for TCC arthrodesis, with the same advantages of the lateral incision, distal fibula removal, and use as a bone graft filling the residual bone defect and voids.[10,21] When the body of the talus is missing, but the neck and/or the head present, the residual talus may be fixed into the anterior tibia after surface preparation, providing a more stable fixation and better chances of a plantigrade foot.[10,21,23] Segmental bone loss (as the talus) is a critical condition, and TC arthrodesis is an attempt to maintain the foot in a plantigrade, stable, and functioning way. The limb is shortened. The surgeon tries to preserve the mobility of the midfoot, but it is not always possible, and sometimes the navicular becomes unstable, and it is unpredictable. In those cases, the midfoot will secondarily deform with weightbearing; this is a limitation of TC arthrodesis, and very few articles discuss what we should do with the navicular in a complete absence of talus in a TC arthrodesis.

The patient in **Fig. 5** had an ankle and hindfoot CN with loss of the talar body. A TC arthrodesis was done, and the residual talar head was prepared (dorsal and plantar faces) to be interposed between the anterior space of tibia and calcaneus. The residual talar segment was too short to provide an adequate stability. The association of Chopart arthrodesis in this case allowed for a better correction and stability.

Metcalf and Ochenjele[21] discussed a case report of a traumatic extrusion of the talus in a non-DM and CN patient. They chose TC arthrodesis to treat this patient and noticed instability of the midfoot after TC fixation during the surgery. The solution was the combination of the calcaneocuboid arthrodesis with a naviculotibial arthrodesis with bone graft. Mirzayan and colleagues[23] treated 7 patients with rigid

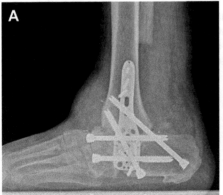
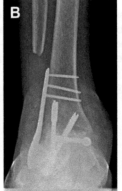
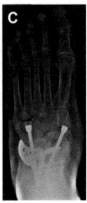

Fig. 5. TC arthrodesis, fixed with locking plate and compression screws. Note that the patient had a residual talar head with body and neck loss. To enhance the stability, we preferred, in this case, to associate a Chopart arthrodesis. (*A–C*) Respectively, radiographs with lateral view and AP view of the ankle and AP of the foot, showing radiographic union.

equinovarus deformity by a total talectomy and TC arthrodesis. In all their cases, to enhance the stability of the fixation, the investigators resected the anterior cortex of the tibia and the articular cartilage of the navicular, fixating them. These 2 articles do not discuss about the deformity nor the fixation in CN but discuss that technically. At least some cases of TC arthrodesis of the calcaneocuboid and tibionavicular joints should be added for better stability and perhaps predictability (**Fig. 6**).

There are other options to treat talar bone loss, as for instance making a TC arthrodesis and filling the voids with graft.

GRAFT

Patients with CN may present with progressive bone loss due to the disease's pathophysiology or the debridement of osteomyelitic bone. For these patients' arthrodesis, a bone graft can be used to restore or maintain the length and to help to stabilize the joint for fusion.[24–26] Also, a graft can promote an increase in vascularization and bone growth factors. The graft can be an autologous, allograft, or bone substitute, depending on the intended function and size of the graft. Autograft has the best biology. It can be cancellous for biology, structural to maintain the length and stability, or vascularized bone graft that has all the previous advantages plus the increase in the blood supply to the region. Nevertheless, each type increases the morbidity of the extraction procedure, which should be a concern, considering these patients tend to have several comorbidities.[24] When the defect is considered too big to use a tricortical structural autograft, a femoral head graft can be used in place. The literature has shown good results for this technique but at the expense of an increased chance of nonunion and nonintegration of the graft.[19,24,27,28] The literature has also started to discuss the use of growth factors to lower the high rate of nonunion in these patients. Hockenbury and colleagues[29] demonstrated a reasonable fusion rate of 90%, with the only patient with nonunion having previously active osteomyelitis of the tibia. Newer studies have shown that the union rate might go up to 97% depending on the growth factor mixed in the bone graft.[30,31] Jeong and colleagues[32] described a case in which a nonvascularized fibula was used as a graft combined with external fixation. In the first approach, the patient was submitted for a TTC arthrodesis using screws and resecting the distal tip of the fibula, a construct that typically does not give the stability that patients with CN need. In this revision, they resected 15 cm of the fibula and used similar to a retrograde intramedullary nail to help create stability through the joints. In

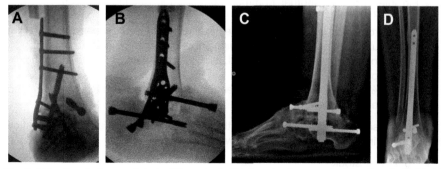

Fig. 6. TC arthrodesis associated with naviculotibial and calcaneocuboid arthrodesis. (*A, B*) AP and lateral radiographs of fixation with locking plate and compression screws; (*C, D*) lateral and AP views of fixation with an intramedullary nail for hindfoot and ankle and compression screws for the Chopart.

their view, the fibula was more biological, which could help increase the chances of union, but there are no other studies to confirm this statement.

EXTERNAL FIXATION

The use of an external fixator to treat CN was first described by Sticha and colleagues[33] in 1996. Although intramedullary nail has become the most popular implant, external fixators may play a role in selected cases. Although some articles describe the use of monoplane external fixator, surgeons usually prefer circular fixators such as Ilizarov or hexapods.[34,35]

The typical indications for external fixation include the following:
- Gradual correction[25,36–39]
  - This is important when the degree of the deformity does not allow full correction in one surgical procedure and needs gradual correction that can be done in the clinic.
- Local soft tissue problem[25,36,38,40]
  - Several of these patients have ulcers or another soft tissue lesion in the foot and ankle region. This construct can help protect the region, allowing easy wound care and facilitating controlling the evolution of a flap.
- Patients with osteomyelitis or active infection on the foot[25,38–41]
  - The external fixator allows the surgeon to make a staged approach to treat local infection or osteomyelitis with the first surgery aimed to stabilize, debride the infected tissue, resect nonviable bone, and fill the void with an antibiotic spacer. Moreover, after controlling the problem, the spacer can be exchanged for a bone graft.
- Allowing early weight-bearing[38,40,41]
  - Most of the investigators agree that it is unnecessary to wait for completed fusion to allow patients to start weight-bearing with the frame, with some of them allowing patients to bear weight from the first day of post-operative surgery.

Although this has been a classic procedure, the rate of complications varies considerably in the literature.
- Nonunion rate has been reported between 33.3% and 85.7%[35,42–45]
  - Most of these patients develop a fibrotic union that allows them to walk[44]
- Pin infection was another common complication ranging between 17% and 50%[35,42–44,46,47]
  - The protocol to wound dressing the pin site and the wires varies along with the literature, with none of them showing superiority with respect to the rest.
  - Most of the cases were superficial, allowing treatment only with antibiotic.
- Broken pin from 13.8% to 25%[44,46]
- From 0% to 18.2% of the patients needed amputation after having been treated with external fixation[35,42–44,46]

A newer use of external fixation is in the hybrid fixation with an internal fixation method. The indications include the following:
- Poor bone stock[26,38,48,49]
- Increase local stability with superconstruct[26,38]

This procedure has a higher complication rate compared with the use of only one of the techniques, but this can be explained because these patients tend to be more complicated before surgery, with a higher rate of ulcers, prior osteomyelitis, significant bone loss, and uncontrolled DM.[34]

SUMMARY

CN is a systemic disease that causes fractures, dislocations, and deformities involving the foot and ankle, resulting in substantial risk of ulceration, infection, and function loss. Early recognition and prevention of collapsing foot and ankle are still the best options for the management of patients with diabetic CN. Once collapse is present, in the acute phase, the use of an off-loading orthosis and antiresorptive medication are recommended. When the deformity is established itself in the end stage — without infection — salvage procedures should be attempted to obtain a functional, pain-free, plantigrade foot and ankle. For a successful arthrodesis procedure, the principles of adequate joint preparation, deformity correction, and soft tissue protection and care are essentials, associated with robust fixation (internal and/or external), use of different biological graft options in segmental losses, and prolonged off-loading.

CLINICS CARE POINTS

- Managing the Charcot hindfoot and ankle needs a multidisciplinary approach.
- Conservative treatments (braces, insoles) may be successful as long as the disease has a good medical control.
- When major deformities are present more stable superconstructs are necessary.
- When poor bone quality or segmental bone loss is present, the use of a graft of good biological quality is essential.
- Tibiotalocalcaneal fusion is the most common surgical procedure for these patients but, in selected cases, talocalcaneal and tibionavicular fusions need to be considered.

DISCLOSURE

The authors have nothing to disclose.

REFERENCES

1. Galhoum AE, Trivedi V, Askar M, et al. Management of ankle charcot neuroarthropathy: a systematic review. J Clin Med 2021;10(24):5923.
2. Sohn MW, Stuck RM, Pinzur M, et al. Lower-extremity amputation risk after charcot arthropathy and diabetic foot ulcer. Diabetes Care 2010;33(1):98–100.
3. Pradana AS, Phatama KY, Mustamsir E, et al. Double posterior lateral plating arthrodesis for charcot ankle: A case series. Ann Med Surg 2021;65:102250.
4. Dodd A, Daniels TR. Charcot Neuroarthropathy of the Foot and Ankle. J Bone Joint Surg 2018;100(8):696–711.
5. Siebachmeyer M, Boddu K, Bilal A, et al. Outcome of one-stage correction of deformities of the ankle and hindfoot and fusion in Charcot neuroarthropathy using a retrograde intramedullary hindfoot arthrodesis nail. Bone Joint J 2015;97-B(1):76–82.
6. Shaikh N, Vaughan P, Varty K, et al. Outcome of limited forefoot amputation with primary closure in patients with diabetes. Bone Joint J 2013;95-B(8):1083–7.

7. Ettinger S, Stukenborg-Colsman C, Plaass C, et al. Tibiocalcaneal arthrodesis as a limb salvage procedure for complex hindfoot deformities. Arch Orthop Trauma Surg 2016;136(4):457–62.

8. Love B, Alexander B, Ray J, et al. Outcomes of tibiocalcaneal arthrodesis in high-risk patients: an institutional cohort of 18 patients. Indian J Orthopaedics 2020; 54(1):14–21.

9. LaPorta GA, Nasser EM, Mulhern JL. Tibiocalcaneal arthrodesis in the high-risk foot. J Foot Ankle Surg 2014;53(6):774–86.

10. Aikawa T, Watanabe K, Matsubara H, et al. Tibiocalcaneal fusion for charcot ankle with severe talar body loss: case report and a review of the surgical literature. J Foot Ankle Surg 2016;55(2):247–51.

11. Callahan R, Juliano P, Aydogan U, et al. Avoiding pitfalls of tibiotalocalcaneal nail malposition with internal rotation axial heel view. Foot & Ankle Specialist 2018; 11(6):543–7.

12. Chraim M, Krenn S, Alrabai HM, et al. Mid-term follow-up of patients with hindfoot arthrodesis with retrograde compression intramedullary nail in Charcot neuro-arthropathy of the hindfoot. Bone Joint J 2018;100-B(2):190–6.

13. Brodsky JW, Rouse AM. Exostectomy for symptomatic bony prominences in diabetic charcot feet. Clin Orthop Relat Res 1993;296:21–6. http://www.ncbi.nlm.nih.gov/pubmed/8222428.

14. Ahmad J, Pour AE, Raikin SM. The Modified Use of a Proximal Humeral Locking Plate for Tibiotalocalcaneal Arthrodesis. Foot Ankle Int 2007;28(9):977–83.

15. Pinzur MS, Kelikian A. Charcot ankle fusion with a retrograde locked intramedullary nail. Foot Ankle Int 1997;18(11):699–704.

16. Paola LD, Volpe A, Varotto D, et al. Use of a retrograde nail for ankle arthrodesis in charcot neuroarthropathy: a limb salvage procedure. Foot Ankle Int 2007;28(9): 967–70.

17. DeVries JG, Berlet GC, Hyer CF. A Retrospective comparative analysis of charcot ankle stabilization using an intramedullary rod with or without application of circular external fixator—utilization of the retrograde arthrodesis intramedullary nail database. J Foot Ankle Surg 2012;51(4):420–5.

18. Caravaggi CMF, Sganzaroli AB, Galenda P, et al. Long-term Follow-up of tibiocalcaneal arthrodesis in diabetic patients with early chronic charcot osteoarthropathy. J Foot Ankle Surg 2012;51(4):408–11.

19. Brandão RA, Weber JS, Larson D, et al. New fixation methods for the treatment of the diabetic foot. Clin Podiatr Med Surg 2018;35(1):63–76.

20. Sammarco VJ. Superconstructs in the treatment of charcot foot deformity: plantar plating, locked plating, and axial screw fixation. Foot Ankle Clin 2009;14(3): 393–407.

21. Metcalf KB, Ochenjele G. Primary triple arthrodesis equivalent for complete extruded missing talus with associated midfoot instability: a case report. JBJS Case Connect 2020;10(2):e0268.

22. Emara KM, Ahmed Diab R, Amr Hemida M. Tibio-calcaneal fusion by retrograde intramedullary nailing in charcot neuroarthropathy. Foot 2018;34:6–10.

23. Mirzayan R, Early SD, Matthys GA, et al. Single-Stage Talectomy and Tibiocalcaneal Arthrodesis as a Salvage of Severe, Rigid Equinovarus Deformity. Foot Ankle Int 2001;22(3):209–13.

24. Short DJ, Zgonis T. Management of osteomyelitis and bone loss in the diabetic charcot foot and ankle. Clin Podiatr Med Surg 2017;34(3):381–7.

25. Conway JD. Charcot salvage of the foot and ankle using external fixation. Foot Ankle Clin 2008;13(1):157–73.

26. Bajuri MY, Ong SL, Das S, et al. Charcot neuroarthropathy: current surgical management and update. A systematic review. Front Surg 2022;9. https://doi.org/10.3389/fsurg.2022.820826.
27. Jeng CL, Campbell JT, Tang EY, et al. Tibiotalocalcaneal arthrodesis with bulk femoral head allograft for salvage of large defects in the ankle. Foot Ankle Int 2013;34(9):1256–66.
28. Ramanujam CL, Facaros Z, Zgonis T. An overview of bone grafting techniques for the diabetic charcot foot and ankle. Clin Podiatr Med Surg 2012;29(4):589–95.
29. Hockenbury RT, Gruttadauria M, McKinney I. Use of implantable bone growth stimulation in charcot ankle arthrodesis. Foot Ankle Int 2007;28(9):971–6.
30. Loveland JD, McMillen RL, Cala MA. A Multicenter, Retrospective, Case Series of Patients With Charcot Neuroarthropathy Deformities Undergoing Arthrodesis Utilizing Recombinant Human Platelet-derived Growth Factor With Beta-Tricalcium Phosphate. J Foot Ankle Surg 2021;60(1):74–9.
31. Pinzur MS. Use of platelet-rich concentrate and bone marrow aspirate in high-risk patients with charcot arthropathy of the foot. Foot Ankle Int 2009;30(02):124–7.
32. Jeong ST, Park HB, Hwang SC, et al. Use of intramedullary nonvascularized fibular graft with external fixation for revisional charcot ankle fusion: a case report. J Foot Ankle Surg 2012;51(2):249–53.
33. Sticha RS, Frascone ST, Wertheimer SJ. Major arthrodeses in patients with neuropathic arthropathy. J Foot Ankle Surg 1996;35(6):560–6.
34. Dayton P, Feilmeier M, Thompson M, et al. Comparison of complications for internal and external fixation for charcot reconstruction: a systematic review. J Foot Ankle Surg 2015;54(6):1072–5.
35. Shah NS, De SD. Comparative analysis of uniplanar external fixator and retrograde intramedullary nailing for ankle arthrodesis in diabetic Charcot's neuroarthropathy. Indian J Orthopaedics 2011;45(4):359–64.
36. Short DJ, Zgonis T. Circular external fixation as a primary or adjunctive therapy for the podoplastic approach of the diabetic charcot foot. Clin Podiatr Med Surg 2017;34(1):93–8.
37. Wrotslavsky P, Kriger SJ, Hammer-Nahman SM, et al. Computer-Assisted Gradual Correction of Charcot Foot Deformities: An In-Depth Evaluation of Stage One of a Planned Two-Stage Approach to Charcot Reconstruction. J Foot Ankle Surg 2020;59(4):841–8.
38. Martin B, Chow J. The use of circular frame external fixation in the treatment of ankle/hindfoot Charcot Neuroarthropathy. J Clin Orthopaedics Trauma 2021;16:269–76.
39. Herbst SA. External fixation of Charcot arthropathy. Foot Ankle Clin 2004;9(3):595–609.
40. Cooper PS. Application of external fixators for management of Charcot deformities of the foot and ankle. Foot Ankle Clin 2002;7(1):207–54.
41. Cates NK, Miller JD, Chen S, et al. Safety of tibial half pins with circular external fixation for foot and ankle reconstruction in patients with peripheral neuropathy. J Foot Ankle Surg 2021. https://doi.org/10.1053/j.jfas.2021.12.021.
42. ElAlfy B, Ali AM, Fawzy SI. Ilizarov external fixator versus retrograde intramedullary nailing for ankle joint arthrodesis in diabetic Charcot neuroarthropathy. J Foot Ankle Surg 2017;56(2):309–13.
43. Richman J, Cota A, Weinfeld S. Intramedullary nailing and external ring fixation for tibiotalocalcaneal arthrodesis in charcot arthropathy. Foot Ankle Int 2017;38(2):149–52.

44. Wirth SH, Viehöfer AF, Tondelli T, et al. Mid-term walking ability after Charcot foot reconstruction using the Ilizarov ring fixator. Arch Orthop Trauma Surg 2020; 140(12):1909–17.
45. Ettinger S, Plaass C, Claassen L, et al. Surgical management of charcot deformity for the foot and ankle—radiologic outcome after internal/external fixation. J Foot Ankle Surg 2016;55(3):522–8.
46. Rogers LC, Bevilacqua NJ, Frykberg RG, et al. Predictors of postoperative complications of ilizarov external ring fixators in the foot and ankle. J Foot Ankle Surg 2007;46(5):372–5.
47. Finkler ES, Kasia C, Kroin E, et al. Pin tract infection following correction of charcot foot with static circular fixation. Foot Ankle Int 2015;36(11):1310–5.
48. Hegewald KW, Wilder ML, Chappell TM, et al. Combined internal and external fixation for diabetic charcot reconstruction: a retrospective case series. J Foot Ankle Surg 2016;55(3):619–27.
49. El-Mowafi H, Abulsaad M, Kandil Y, et al. Hybrid fixation for ankle fusion in diabetic charcot arthropathy. Foot Ankle Int 2018;39(1):93–8.

Tibiotalocalcaneal Arthrodesis in Severe Hindfoot Deformities

Pilar Martínez-de-Albornoz, MD, PhD[a,b,*],
Manuel Monteagudo, MD[a,b]

KEYWORDS

- Ankle • Arthritis • Allograft • Retrograde nail • Treatment • Arthrodesis • Deformity
- Tibiotalocalcaneal arthrodesis

KEY POINTS

- Many patients with end-stage ankle/hindfoot arthritis and severe deformity present with previous sequelae (nonunion, malunion, broken implants, vascular deficiencies, skin problems).
- Surgical planning needs to be very detailed and thorough with a special focus on bone loss after debridement of non-healthy tissue and removal of metalwork.
- The surgical approach should be individualized and largely depends on the soft-tissue envelope of previous scars and vascular studies.
- Tibiotalocalcaneal arthrodesis (TTCA) with grafting is the most common and reliable procedure in the treatment of patients with end-stage ankle arthritis combined with severe deformity.
- Although most patients are satisfied with their outcome, nonunion rates of around 20% of cases and around 5% of cases will end in an amputation.

INTRODUCTION

Severe hindfoot and ankle deformities are usually the end-stage result of a severe initial injury and sometimes suboptimal subsequent surgeries ending up in an unbraceble and dysfunctional foot with untreatable severe pain. More than 70% of severely deformed arthritic ankles are post-traumatic (rotational ankle fractures), with 30% being caused by inflammatory or primary arthritis.[1] These patients frequently present with instability and multiple scars and had suffered previous skin problems and/or infection, stiffness, and changes in the biomechanics of several joints around the foot and ankle. Frail

The authors have nothing to disclose.
[a] Orthopaedic Foot and Ankle Unit, Orthopaedic and Trauma Department, Hospital Universitario Quirónsalud, Madrid, Spain; [b] Faculty Medicine UEM, Madrid, Spain
* Corresponding author.
E-mail address: pilarmalbornoz@hotmail.com

patients with fragile bones are in special risk of ending up with deformed arthritic ankles. Broken metalwork, extensive bone loss, and vascular impairment are also present in many of these complex cases. The subgroup of patients that we will consider in this article are not candidates for joint-preservation realignment osteotomies nor for total ankle replacement because of extensive chondral damage and severe deformity. We will not cover severe deformities in Charcot cases (Chapter 8).

When all conservative treatments fail to alleviate pain and dysfunction, arthrodeses are the procedure of choice for hindfoot/ankle arthritis with severe deformity. Tibiotalo-calcaneal arthrodesis (TTCA) is one of the most common procedures to be considered for these patients.[2] Some of these patients have already undergone repeated failed surgeries and amputation is another alternative to yet another reconstructive intervention. Indeed, some patients directly ask for an amputation exhausted after a long fight against all odds. Recent advances in technical issues in the field of lower limb prosthetics have closed the gap between complex reconstruction versus below-the-knee amputation.

In cases with an established indication of a new salvage procedure, TTCA frequently has to deal with the need to bone graft and include adjacent joint to achieve a pantalar fusion. Whenever the Chopart joint is flexible and not severely damaged it should be preserved to allow motion in the sagittal plane to compensate for the loss of hindfoot and ankle motion after TTCA.[3] Valgus positioning of the TTCA is paramount to allow for potential maximized compensatory motion around the midtarsal joints.[4]

The aim of the present article is bringing the reader up to the understanding of complex cases with severe deformity and discuss about the indication of TTCA, the mechanics after the procedure, the surgical planning and technique with tips and tricks, the results with complications and outcomes, and the rationale after considering TTCA as a potential better indication than amputation.

EVALUATION AND MANAGEMENT OF SEVERE HINDFOOT DEFORMITIES

Most of these patients have already undergone several surgeries and a wide array of conservative interventions. It is fundamental to study all previous procedures to address the estate of the patient and the regional scenario comprising the skin, soft-tissues, bone quality, and stock. A thorough clinical examination and additional metabolic (Hemoglobin A1c), vascular, and image studies are necessary to delimitate the extent of arthritis and study factors that might condition decision-making during the preoperative planning. Image studies should include weightbearing X-rays of both feet and ankles, computed tomography, and magnetic resonance. Infections and diabetic patients will be covered in another chapter.

CONSERVATIVE TREATMENT

Although conservative treatment should always be attempted before indicating surgery, most of these patients are difficult to brace and to adapt to any orthoses. Rehabilitation therapies have usually a low impact in the quality of life of this population.[5] While trying to alleviate pain with non-operative treatments, patient general health condition should be optimized if possible.

SURGICAL TREATMENT

TTCA with an intramedullary hindfoot nail is an established and the most popular procedure for fusion of the ankle and subtalar joints.[6] In cases involving ankle bone loss, such as in failed total ankle replacement, it can be difficult to salvage with sufficient bone restoration stability and a physiologic leg length to avoiding below-the-knee amputation. In the last years, failure of ankle arthrodesis or total ankle replacement is a more common scenario in our practice and results in a challenging clinical situation.[7] It may take the form of septic revision or a big bone defect after aseptic loosening of the implants. Arthrodesis following a failed Total ankle replacement (TAR) is almost invariably a TTCA as the subtalar joint is usually arthritic and/or there is significant bone loss from the talus (**Fig. 1**). Revision in these setting is technically demanding, and if associated with subtalar degeneration, conversion to TTCA may be required, with use of bone grafting to maintain length and reduce disability.[7] TTCA is also indicated when poor bone stock is present in the talus because of avascular necrosis or in cases of

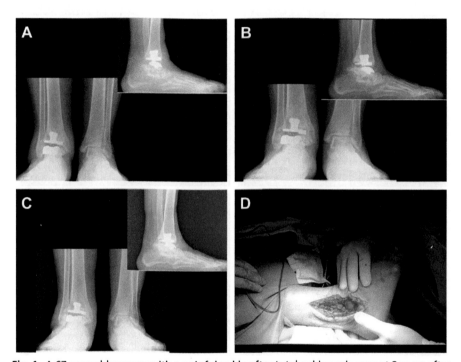

Fig. 1. A 67-year-old woman with a painful ankle after total ankle replacement 2 years after surgery. (*A*) Weight-bearing radiographs showing suboptimal positioning of the components. (*B*) 6 months later, a progressive collapse of the talar component was evident. (*C*) One year from the first X-rays shown, collapse and displacement affected both the tibial and talar components. The patient was very symptomatic at this stage. (*D*) Intraoperative view of tibiotalocalcaneal arthrodesis with femoral head to fill the ankle defect after the removal of implants. (*E*) Iliac crest autograft allowed for the filling of the voids after allograft. (*F*) Postoperative radiographs after revision surgery to tibiotalocalcaneal arthrodesis with retrograde nailing. (*G*) Weight-bearing radiographs 12 months after nailing. The patient suffered hindfoot pain and she was diagnosed of symptomatic subtalar nonunion with a fused tibiotalar. (*H*) Revision surgery included nail removal, preparation of subtalar joint and screw fixation t 6 months from surgery the ankle remained painful and showed signs of nonunion. (*I*) New revision surgery consisting in tibiotalocalcaneal arthrodesis with more iliac crest grafting and tiobiotalocalcaneal plate. (*J*) One year after the last procedure, the patient was pain-free, and the anteroposterior weight-bearing radiographs showed solid fusion with a correct valgus position. (*K*) Lateral view of the fused tibiotalocalcaneal joints. (*L*) The patient was very satisfied with outcome but at the expense of considerable shortening of the operated leg.

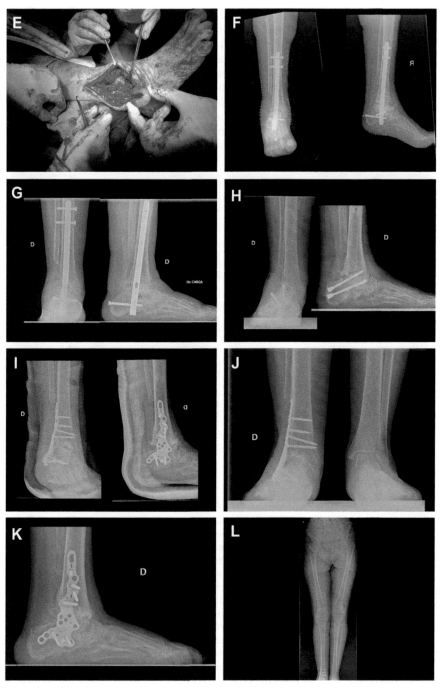

Fig. 1. (*continued*).

severe deformity, and poor soft-tissue conditions. All these scenarios are common when dealing with complex challenging cases. Surgical planning is essential in these complex cases.

SURGICAL TECNIQUE

The ideal position for TTCA is plantigrade with the hindfoot 0° to 5° of valgus, 5° to 10° of external rotation and the talus posteriorly translated under the tibia. Coronal alignment should allow about 5° of hindfoot valgus, which may be achieved directly when fixing the subtalar.[4] The tibiotalar and subtalar surfaces should be as well-apposed as possible and moderate compression should be achieved with the use of screws, nail, or lateral plate and screws. Postoperatively the ankle has been traditionally kept nonweightbearing for approximately 4 to 6 weeks and weight bearing is initiated as tolerated in a protective walker boot.

The to-do-list in the planning of surgery include:

1. Surgical approach.
2. Bone stock-grafting.
3. Implants.
4. The fibula.
5. Joints around the ankle/hindfoot.

Surgical Approach

Surgical approach for the correction of a big hindfoot/ankle deformity may be conditioned by previous metalwork, previous approaches, skin status, and vascular status of the patient. A variety of operative approaches have been described for TTCA.[8] Lateral transfibular approach was first developed to allow for direct and quick access to both tibiotalar and subtalar joints. But many patients present with previous lateral scars and a thin skin envelope. Medial, posterolateral, and posterior (Achilles tendon-splitting) approaches are available as alternatives to the more conventional lateral approach. Patients should ideally undergo a vascular evaluation to map potential compromised areas of poor blood supply that might condition the approach and compromise the soft-tissues in the postoperative period (**Fig. 2**).

Lateral (transfibular) approach: Hess and colleagues[9] studied this approach for different indications and techniques, with focus on postoperative outcomes among procedures performed. For TTCA, the rate of deep infection was 3.7% (4 of 106) concluding that the transfibular approach yields satisfactory results, with low complication and infection rates (**Fig. 3**).

Posterior (Achilles tendon-splitting) approach: It offers a well-vascularized, thick, soft-tissue envelope. Several authors have described technical details on the combination of posterior approach to the tibiotalar and subtalar joints with good exposure for resection and deformity correction in TTCA.[10,11] Grafting, posterior tibiotalocalcaneal plates, and nails can be used in combination with the posterior approach with comparable good results.[12] The largest series of TTCA fusions via posterior Achilles tendon-splitting approach studied 41 patients with an intramedullary TTC nail used in 37 patients (90.2%), with posterior plate or supplemental screw augmentation in 17 patients.[13] Posterior plate fixation alone was used in 4 cases (9.8%). Union rate was 80.4% and complications included 17 patients included ankle nonunion (19.5%), tibial stress fracture (17%), postoperative cellulitis and superficial wound breakdown (9.7%), subtalar nonunion (4.8%), and malunion (2.4%). One patient eventually underwent amputation (2.4%). Mulligan and colleagues[14] compared the results

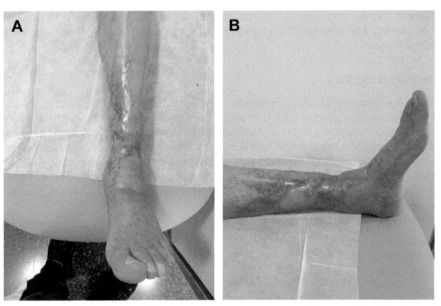

Fig. 2. Skin and soft-tissue problems are common among candidates to tibiotalocalcaneal arthrodesis. (*A*) Multiple scars and flap coverage after several surgeries. (*B*) The condition of soft-tissues around the ankle and hindfoot may condition the surgical approach for the arthrodesis.

of TTCA with a posterior approach with nailing in 38 patients versus lateral approach with fixed-angle plating in 28 patients. All cases were complex, and the overall union rate was 71%; 76% (29 of 38 patients) for posterior approach with nailing, and 64% (18 of 28) for the lateral approach with plating. There were no significant differences in results nor in complications, so the authors conclude both procedures are adequate when dealing with different scenarios (prior incisions, preexisting metalwork, deformity).

Other approaches: Rausch and colleagues[8] studied the effects of 3 approaches (lateral transfibular, medial, and posterolateral) on the neurovascular structures and quantified the extent of cartilage in the different joints that could be surgically debrided in 12 specimens. Transfibular approach had less risk of damaging arteries, whereas the posterolateral approach was particularly likely to damage the lateral malleolar branches of the peroneal artery. Medial approach was the most risk-bearing of the

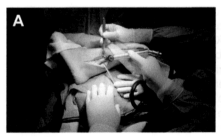
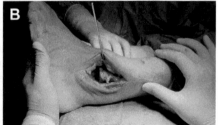

Fig. 3. Lateral transfibular approach allows for a direct and quick access to the ankle and subtalar joints. (*A*) Fibular osteotomy. (*B*) Intraoperative view of the tibiotalar joint after lateral approach.

3 approaches in terms of venous structures and nerve damage. The proportions of cartilage-debrided joint surfaces did not differ notably.

Although in the last few years arthroscopic ankle arthrodesis and mini-invasive osteotomies and arthrodesis have gained popularity, most of our complex deformed cases will need a big approach with grafting, a good final correction/alignment, and the choice of an implant that allows for the maximum mechanical primary stability to achieve solid union at the arthrodesis site. However, there is a subset of patients with previous skin breakdowns and infections in which a minimally invasive (non-arthroscopic) may allow for a safer TTCA. Carranza-Bencano and colleagues[15] reported on a big series of 40 patients that underwent minimally invasive (non-arthroscopic) TTCA achieving bony union in 86% of cases.60 In selected cases with end-stage arthritis but moderate deformity, arthroscopic TTCA drastically reduced infections with the same union rates as conventional open TTC.[16] Baumbach and colleagues[17] compared arthroscopic to open TTCA in high-risk patients. Eight open and 15 arthroscopic cases were evaluated. Fusion rates were similar (75% vs 67%) and major complications occurred in 63% of open (80% surgical-site-infections) and 33% of arthroscopic (100% nonunions) TTCA.

Bone Stock: Grafting

In most complex cases of ankle/hindfoot arthritis with deformity It is common to encounter a large bony void that needs to be filled with grafting. This is specially the case of revision surgery following a failed total ankle replacement. Large osseous defects of the hindfoot and ankle are a surgical challenge. Femoral head allografts are frequently used to achieve fusion and preserve limb length, but these structural allografts can be challenging because of their inherent poor healing capacity, with fusion rates reported as low as 50% when a femoral head allograft was used with an intramedullary nail.[18,19]

Femoral head allografts: In a systematic review on the use of structural allograft in patients undergoing TTCA, Cifaldi and colleagues[20] evaluated rates of union, limb salvage and complications. In a total of 11 publications with 175 patients, femoral head allograft was the most used structural graft, and a retrograde intramedullary nail was the most common fixation construct. Overall union rate was 67.4%, with a complication rate of 26.6%. There was no significant difference in union rate when using a nail versus a plate construct. Despite high rates of radiographic nonunion, patients avoided amputation in over 90% of cases. In another study, Coetzee and colleagues[21] reported the results of 44 patients that underwent TTCA using a femoral head allograft. All patients had either failure of primary or revision total ankle arthroplasty or avascular necrosis of the talus. Union rate reached 90.7% of the ankles with five patients needing revision surgery for symptomatic nonunions. Patient satisfaction was high. Jeng and colleagues[22] also used bulk femoral head allograft to fill large segmental bony defects after different failed surgeries. Thirty-two patients underwent TTCA with allografting resulting in 50% of unions with 19% of the patients requiring a below-the-knee amputation. Diabetes mellitus was found to be the only predictive factor of bad outcome.

Graft preparation: Femoral heads from bone banks are prepared to fit into the defect (**Fig. 4**). The use of acetabular reamers helps to create a concave surface for placement of a convex femoral head allograft. This "cup-and-cone" ("ball-in-basket") technique provides a congruent area for the allograft, with enhanced stability of the graft during placement of an intramedullary nail.[23–25]

Trabecular metal. Extended bone loss around the ankle has been associated with high rates of nonunion and shortening of the limb because of graft resorption or

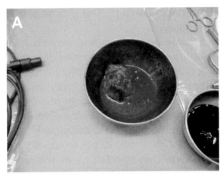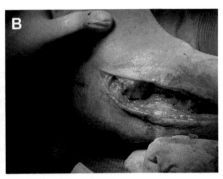

Fig. 4. Grafting in revision surgery for tibiotalocalcaneal arthrodesis is a common necessity. (A) Femoral head ready to be implanted to fit into a big ankle defect. (B) After the insertion of the femoral head into the defect, the surgeon should consider other void fillers for the remaining joint space.

collapse.[26] Trabecular metal interpositional spacers have been specifically designed for TTCA with nailing. These spacers can be implanted using either an anterior or a lateral approach. An integrated hole allows for the insertion of a retrograde nail, apparently providing good primary stability of the construct.[26] Although good results have been reported with small series of patients,[26–28] Aubret and colleagues[29] reported disappointing results at 1-year follow-up in 11 patients with 5 patients showing lack of tantalum integration and symptomatic nonunion. The development of 3-dimensional printed titanium trusses has given surgeons an alternative to allografts by providing structural support to prevent collapse.[30,31]

Other void fillers and adjuncts: Sherman and colleagues[32] used adjunctive osteoinductive agents and prolonged protected weightbearing to assess potential improvements of outcomes with respect to the conventional technique. Fourteen patients underwent bone block TTCA biologically augmented with fresh-frozen femoral head allograft, bone marrow aspirate concentrate, and demineralized bone matrix cortical fibers. Fusion was documented on plain radiograph in 13 of 14 patients (92.9%) and CT in 10 of 11 patients (90.9%). One patient (7.1%) experienced nonunion and persistent infection requiring amputation. In the same study, three patients underwent a vascularized reconstruction with a medial femoral condyle free flap with shorter time to fusion. Suboptimal results reported with structural block allografts in TTCA led other surgeons to use distal tibial structural allograft to obtain a more stable TTC fusion. Escudero and colleagues[33] evaluated 10 patients with prior nonunion after failed total ankle arthroplasties. Union rate was 80%. In seven cases the allograft did not lose height. A lower rate of collapse than other structural grafts provided a fusion rate higher or similar to other studies using femoral head allograft. Vaughn and colleagues[34] attempted a novel technique using fresh allograft talus in attempt to improve nonunion rate in TTCA. Five patients obtained fusion, including two diabetic patients and two former smokers. There were no complications and functional outcomes were encouraging. Rabiu and colleagues[35] developed a sliding oblique hindfoot osteotomy as an alternative to bulk allografts. The oblique osteotomy was performed to correct anterior talus subluxation and prevent excessive loss of height at the tibiotalar apposition and to correct the varus-valgus deformity. A retrograde hindfoot nail was used in 9 patients. All patients went on to fusion and were ambulating at 6 months. All were satisfied with the outcome of their treatment.

Implants

Implant selection may be conditioned by the surgical approach, the need for bone grafting, previous infection, or previous metalwork. The choice of implants and type of grafting largely depends on the surgeon's preference and experience, but also on the alignment of the ankle, quality of bone stock, soft-tissue conditions, surgical approach, risk factors, and patient expectations.

Nails

Retrograde interlocking nailing represents one of the biomechanically most stable fixation methods after reconstruction of hindfoot alignment. Over the years, nail designs have adapted to the tibiotalocalcaneal geometry and incorporated sustained compression across fusion sites and posterior-to-anterior locking providing good mechanical primary stability (**Figs. 5** and **6**). Incorporation of compression has apparently been a big improvement for the outcome of retrograde nailing. Some studies reported that patients treated with second-generation nails incorporating an internal compression mechanism experienced faster times to fusion and higher fusion rates than patients treated with first-generation nails lacking an internal compression feature.[36,37] Compression has been shown to be important not only in stabilizing the arthrodesis sites but also in promoting bone healing at a faster speed and allowing for load sharing between implanted devices and native osseous tissue to prevent fatigue fracture of hardware.[19,36–38]

Several authors have reported on patients with severe hindfoot/ankle deformities that underwent TTCA with retrograde nailing.[39–41] The overall union rate was approximately 80% with approximately 20% of patients needing revision surgery for nonunion, malunion, infection or amputation. Nails have also evolved toward different shapes and designs to better adapt to the complex anatomy of the tibiotalocalcaneal region. New nails seem to improve overall results for fusion.[42,43] Augmentation with a screw in TTCA with intramedullary nail fixation, provided more stable fixation, particularly in patients with osteopenic bone.[44]

Plates (and/or Screws)

Blade plates have traditionally been used for TTCA. Some authors have demonstrated high rates of union when using blade plates.[14,45–47] Chodos and colleagues[48] reported that fixation with a locking plate was superior to that of a blade plate. To improve nonunion and revision rates obtained with nails and blade plates, specifically designed TTCA locking plates have been developed with a better matching between irregular bone and implants.[49] Several specific tibiotalocalcaneal plates are now available for lateral and posterior fixation of a TTCA (**Fig. 7**).

Comparison between different implants: Several authors have compared the use of nails and plates for TTCA. In a cadaveric study, Alfahd and colleagues[50] found no significant differences between plates and nails. Some authors have suggested that there was no rotational biomechanical advantage of an intramedullary nail when compared with blade plate fixation in a cadaveric TTCA model regardless bone mineral density.[51] Hamid and colleagues[52] evaluated compressive forces at the ankle and subtalar joints with 3 partially threaded cannulated screws, hindfoot nail, and lateral plate. Lateral TTCA plates provided increased compressive forces at the ankle and subtalar joint compared with screws-only constructs. Hindfoot nails did not demonstrate significant differences in either of these parameters compared with plates or screws in this study. Bennet and colleagues biomechanically tested the stability and micromotion in four methods of fixation: three crossed 6.5-mm cancellous screws, two crossed 6.5-mm

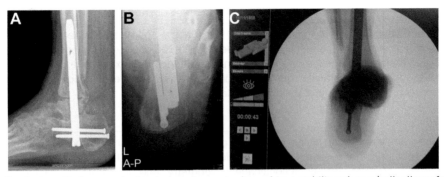

Fig. 5. A meticulous surgical technique is required to achieve stability when a bulk allograft is used for tibiotalocalcaneal arthrodesis. (*A*) Lateral standing view showing signs of nonunion after a tibiotalocalcaneal arthrodesis with a nail and femoral head allograft. (*B*) Axial view shows a potential cause for failure. Distal postero-to-anterior locking screws are not passing through the nail. (*C*) Fluoroscopic control of the posterior-to-anterior screws is advised to avoid the abovementioned complication.

cancellous screws, locked retrograde intramedullary rod, and locked retrograde intramedullary rod augmented with a single anteromedial bone staple. Biomechanically, a staple augmented locked intramedullary rod conferred excellent stability nearly equal to the three crossed cancellous screw technique. Some authors found plating superior to nailing when performing TTCA.[53,54] All TTCA plating systems still have to be evaluated in patients but given their recent availability, it will still take time to be sure that cadaveric studies result in the same outcomes than studies in patients with a minimum follow up.

External Fixation

In cases of severe misalignment, poor bone stock, and critical soft-tissue conditions and/or poor perfusion an external fixation may be contemplated (**Fig. 8**). Reports on the outcomes of the Ilizarov ring or comparable external fixation techniques for ankle fusion are rare, with the ones available accounting for fusion rates between 80% and 100%.[55,56] External fixators are widely used in Charcot patients.

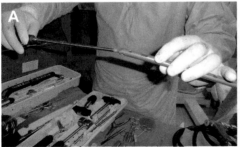
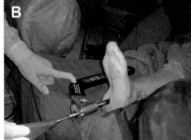

Fig. 6. Compression through the tibiotalar and subtalar joints has allowed new nails to improve overall union rates in tibiotalocalcaneal arthrodesis. (*A*) Preloading of the tibiotalar screw into the nail before insertion. (*B*) Use of the compression screwdriver for the preloaded screw to achieve good apposition between the tibia and talus.

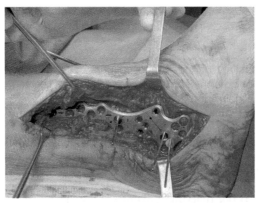

Fig. 7. A tibiotalocalcaneal plate is used via lateral transfibular approach after nonunion with a nail.

The Fibula

Lateral approach to the ankle and hindfoot requires a fibular osteotomy to gain adequate access to the tibiotalar and subtalar joints. Commonly, the distal part of the fibula is not used for the rest of the procedure. Sometimes the cancellous bone within the distal fibula is harvested to fill voids in the prepared joints for fusion. Some other authors use the fibula for autografting.

Circular pillar augmentation with fibular autografting has been indicated in combination with a TTC retrograde nail, an anterior plate, and structural allograft for cases with severe ankle bone loss and instability.[57,58] An *intramedullary fibular structural graft* has been used in complex cases to improve union rates in TTCA.[59] After fibular osteotomy and joint preparation, the fibular strut graft was introduced intramedullary and an external fixator or plate and screws were used for fixation. Sixteen patients underwent TTCA with this procedure and 13 achieved union. Thirteen patients (81.2%) subsequently achieved union.

In cases of recalcitrant nonunion after TTCA or poor biology and regional vascular supply, the use of a vascularized pedicled fibular onlay bone graft could be an alternative procedure. Roukis and colleagues[60] presented good results in 10 cases of TTCA with this technique. Watanabe[61] presented a technique to fill a large bone defect

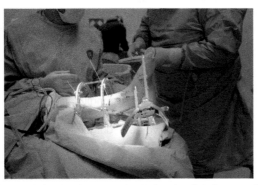

Fig. 8. Active recalcitrant infection is a common indication for the use of an external fixator for tibiotalocalcaneal arthrodesis.

using a soft-tissue-preserved fibular strut graft and obtained fusion in all cases, possibly because of preserving blood supply to the fibular graft.

The Subtalar Joint

TTCA with intramedullary nailing in conventional cases is usually performed with formal preparation of both the subtalar and ankle joints. There is controversy about whether the subtalar joint preparation is necessary to achieve satisfactory results. Although some authors have reported a similar decline in pain, with a high rate of union, and a decrease in operative time when the subtalar joint was not prepared,[62] most studies suggest that subtalar joint preparation should usually be performed in complex deformities because there is a need for axial correction via intraarticular wedge-shaped osteotomies to realign the hindfoot and ankle.[63,64]

PATHOMECHANICS AFTER TIBIOTALOCALCANEAL ARTHRODESIS

In patients presenting with end-stage arthritis and severe deformity of the foot and ankle the goal of a reconstructive procedure is to achieve a painless ankle and foot while preserving motion and gait parameters as close to a healthy limb as possible. Stability is more important than motion in this setting although joints around the arthrodesis should ideally be as mobile as possible. When the subtalar joint is fixed in slight valgus, the midtarsal joints would adapt by increasing their sagittal motion and compensate the loss of sagittal motion in the ankle-subtalar complex.[3] This may explain why patients after TTCA show an even greater increase in midfoot load.[65] In a TTCA we may effectively fix the subtalar in slight valgus thus influencing the adaptation of the midtarsal joints compensation. Different studies comparing gait in TTCA versus tibiotalar arthrodesis demonstrate similar results with no differences were found in terms of pain, satisfaction, and return to work.[66]

RESULTS/COMPLICATIONS/OUTCOMES

Although historical series reported high rates of nonunion, infection, and amputation after TTCA, recent studies presented good functional outcomes with low complication rates. In general, major complications are nonunion, malunions, limb shortening, adjacent joint arthritis and amputation.[67,68] Newer implants specifically built for TCCA have made the procedure easier for the surgeon and more reliable for the patient. Patients scheduled for a revision ankle/hindfoot surgery with severe deformity should know preoperatively that they will never recover a "normal limb" and that any major complication could possibly lead to an amputation.

Complication rates of TTPA are reported to be as high as 40%, with potential nonunion rates over 20%, when indications are made in high-risk patients.[18] Patients in TTC studies have more comorbidities and risk factors for failure than those in primary ankle procedures.[69] Diabetes, diabetic neuropathy, high (>2) American Society of Anesthesiologists (ASA) classification, and Charcot neuroarthropathy—popular among TTC studies—all were predictive of developing a nonunion in the subtalar or tibiotalar joints.[18] Prior peripheral neuropathic conditions have strong evidence for failure to achieve union.[68] Different studies in which osteoarthritis was the main indication for TTC patients reported more favorable outcomes with union rates close to 100%.[19,70] Some authors have presented good results after TTCA, with 50% of patients not being handicapped in the performance of daily activities and 44% being in the same job as at the time of injury.[18,71,72] Levinson and colleagues[69] highlighted the high complication rate after studying 47 cases with successful fusion of 79% for the tibiotalar, 70% for the subtalar, and 66% for combined tibiotalar and subtalar

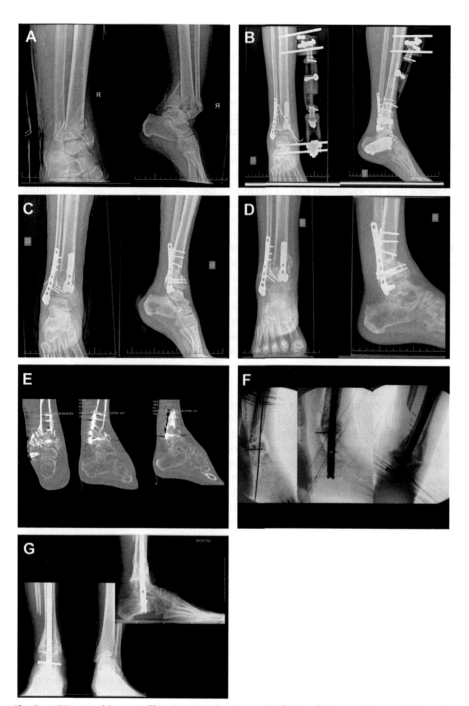

Fig. 9. A 37-year-old man suffered a pilon fracture with fibular fracture after a vehicle crash. (*A*) Initial radiographs showing severe comminution and displacement. (*B*) Initial surgery combined external and internal fixation. (*C*) External fixation was removed 3 months after index surgery and suboptimal reduction is now evident. (*D*) Progressive deformity and

joints. Eight of 47 (17%) TTC nails suffered nail breakage postoperatively. The authors suggested improvements in implant design to decrease revision rates and improve outcomes. Mehta and colleagues[73] used Patient-Reported Outcome Measurement Information System (PROMIS) Physical Function (PF) and Pain Interference (PI) Computer Adaptive Tests (CATs) to retrospectively study outcomes after TTCA in 102 patients to conclude that outcomes were favorable in most cases. Different authors[68,70] have analyzed large series of TTCA in search of the relationships between preoperative conditions and postoperative complications trying to predict outcomes following primary TTCA and concluded that Charcot or non-traumatic arthropathy had an increased risk of nonunion and postoperative infection compared with individuals with traumatic arthritis. Patients with diabetes, chronic kidney disease, or aged over 60 years had an increased risk of nonunion. Several authors[74–79] studied the outcomes and complications of patients undergoing TTCA with a femoral nail. Overall clinical union rate was approximately 80% with approximately 5% needing a proximal amputation. Overall complication rate reached 55% of cases in some studies (**Fig. 9**).[13,80] Most patients are satisfied with the results of these salvage operations, and most are able to return to their daily activities and some to their previous work, with statistics that are comparable to satisfaction after below-the-knee amputations.[81] The studies presented in this article have a considerable wide array of different scenarios that obviously bias some of the results, complications, and outcomes but together they present a persuasive pattern toward considering TTC with grafting and nail or plate fixation as a good salvage procedure that may help the patients to maintain their foot and ankle with a better alignment, function, and pain relief.

SUMMARY

TTCA is the most common and reliable procedure in the treatment of patients with end-stage ankle arthritis combined with severe deformity. Many of these patients present with difficult previous sequelae that include nonunion, malunion, broken implants, vascular deficiencies, skin problems, or a combination of the previous. In that complex scenario, sometimes the only alternative treatment is a below-the-knee amputation. Image studies—weightbearing X-rays, tomography, and magnetic resonance—are fundamental to evaluate alignment and bone stock. When all conservative treatments fail to alleviate pain and dysfunction, the combination of osteotomies and arthrodesis is the procedure of choice. Surgical planning needs to be very detailed and thorough with a special focus in bone loss after debridement of non-healthy tissue and removal of metalwork. TTCA with grafting allows for the preservation of the limb in more than 80% of cases but at the expense of many complications with nonunion rates of approximately 20% of cases. There is controversy about the use of a retrograde nail versus specific TTCA plate and screws but results from biomechanical studies do not show a clear superiority of one specific construct. Amputation rates are close to 5% of cases after repeated failed surgeries. Bulk allografts increase the rate of

---

broken metalwork clearly suggest nonunion. (*E*) Tomography confirms nonunion and some nonviable bone in the ankle joint. Subtalar also showed subtle arthritic changes and was symptomatic. (*F*) Fluoroscopic intraoperative images with a distal tibia allograft to fill the big bone defect in the ankle. Iliac crest allograft and retrograde nailing to try to achieve tibiotalocalcaneal arthrodesis. (*G*) One year from the arthrodesis surgery, weight-bearing radiographs demonstrate solid union and graft incorporation and remodeling. The patient was very satisfied and return to his previous work as a fishmonger.

nonunions but apparently do not have an influence on postoperative infections. Valgus positioning of the ankle/hindfoot is paramount to allow for maximal sagittal plane compensation from the midtarsal joints. Most patients are satisfied with the results of these salvage operations. The studies presented in this paper have a considerable wide array of different scenarios that obviously bias some of the results, complications, and outcomes but together they present a persuasive pattern toward considering TTC with grafting and nail or plate fixation as a good salvage procedure that may help the patients to maintain their foot and ankle with a better alignment, function, and pain relief.

CLINICS CARE POINTS

- Tibiotalocalcaneal arthrodesis is the most common and reliable procedure in the treatment of patients with end stage ankle arthritis combined with severe deformity.

- Complex cases need an experienced surgeon as many of these patients require an individualize surgical approach, removal of previous metalwork, grafting, and the use of specific implants to achieve a functional foot/ankle with pain relief.

- Obviously, these scenarios are not free of complications with rates of nonunion of approximately 20% of cases. Not all nonunions are symptomatic though and ankle/hindfoot stability combined with valgus positioning usually results in improvement of gait and overall quality of life.

- Following these complex salvage surgeries, amputations are finally needed in approximately 5% of patients.

- Satisfaction is high in most cases with most patients returning to their daily activities and some to their previous work.

REFERENCES

1. Ewalefo SO, Dombrowski M, Hirase T, et al. Management of Posttraumatic Ankle Arthritis: Literature Review. Curr Rev Musculoskelet Med 2018;11(4):546–57.
2. Asomugha EU, Den Hartog BD, Junko JT, et al. Tibiotalocalcaneal Fusion for Severe deformity and bone loss. J Am Acad Orthop Surg 2016;24(3):125–34.
3. Maceira E, Monteagudo M. Subtalar anatomy and mechanics. Foot Ankle Clin 2015;20(2):195–221.
4. Monteagudo M, Martínez de Albornoz P. TTC vs Deciding Between Ankle and Tibiotalocalcaneal Arthrodesis for Isolated Ankle. Arthritis Foot Ankle Clin 2022; 27(1):217–31.
5. Bloch B, Srinivasan S, Mangwani J. Current Concepts in the Management of Ankle Osteoarthritis: A Systematic Review. J Foot Ankle Surg 2015;54(5):932–9.
6. Kim C, Catanzariti AR, Mendicino RW. Tibiotalocalcaneal arthrodesis for salvage of severe ankle degeneration. Clin Podiatr Med Surg 2009;26(2):283–302.
7. Hopgood P, Kumar R, Wood PL. Ankle arthrodesis for failed total ankle replacement. J Bone Joint Surg Br 2006;88(8):1032–8.
8. Rausch S, Loracher C, Fröber R, et al. Anatomical evaluation of different approaches for tibiotalocalcaneal arthrodesis. Foot Ankle Int 2014;35(2):163–7.
9. Hess MC, Abyar E, McKissack HM, et al. Applications of the transfibular approach to the hindfoot: A systematic review and description of a preferred technique. Foot Ankle Surg 2021;27(1):1–9.

10. Asunción J, Poggio D. Abordaje posterior de tobillo para la artrodesis tibioastragalocalcánea con clavo intramedular retrógrado. Rev Pie Tobillo 2010;24(1):35–47.
11. Didomenico LA, Sann P. Posterior approach using anterior ankle arthrodesis locking plate for tibiotalocalcaneal arthrodesis. J Foot Ankle Surg 2011;50(5):626–9.
12. Eckholt S, Garcia-Elvira R, Fontecilla N, et al. Role of Extra-articular Tibiotalocalcaneal Arthrodesis and Posterior Approach in Highly Complex Cases. Foot Ankle Int 2018;39(2):219–25.
13. Pellegrini MJ, Schiff AP, Adams SB Jr, et al. Outcomes of Tibiotalocalcaneal Arthrodesis Through a Posterior Achilles Tendon-Splitting Approach. Foot Ankle Int 2016;37(3):312–9.
14. Mulligan RP, Adams SB Jr, Easley ME, et al. Comparison of Posterior Approach With Intramedullary Nailing Versus Lateral Transfibular Approach With Fixed-Angle Plating for Tibiotalocalcaneal Arthrodesis. Foot Ankle Int 2017;38(12):1343–51.
15. Carranza-Bencano A, Tejero S, Del Castillo-Blanco G, et al. Minimal incision surgery for tibiotalocalcaneal arthrodesis. Foot Ankle Int 2014;35(3):272–84.
16. Vilá y Rico J, Rodriguez-Martin J, Parra-Sanchez G, et al. Arthroscopic tibiotalocalcaneal arthrodesis with locked retrograde compression nail. J Foot Ankle Surg 2013;52(4):523–8.
17. Baumbach SF, Massen FK, Hörterer S, et al. Comparison of arthroscopic to open tibiotalocalcaneal arthrodesis in high-risk patients. Foot Ankle Surg 2019;25(6):804–11.
18. Kowalski C, Stauch C, Callahan R, et al. Prognostic risk factors for complications associated with tibiotalocalcaneal arthrodesis with a nail. Foot Ankle Surg 2020;26(6):708–11.
19. Lee BH, Fang C, Kunnasegaran R, et al. Tibiotalocalcaneal Arthrodesis With the Hindfoot Arthrodesis Nail: A Prospective Consecutive Series From a Single Institution. J Foot Ankle Surg 2018;57(1):23–30.
20. Cifaldi A, Thompson M, Abicht B. Tibiotalocalcaneal Arthrodesis with Structural Allograft for Management of Large Osseous Defects of the Hindfoot and Ankle: A Systematic Review and Meta-Analysis. J Foot Ankle Surg 2022;61(4):900–6.
21. Coetzee ster LM, Saltzman CL, Leupold J, et al. Long-term results following ankle arthrodesis for post-traumatic arthritis. J Bone Joint Surg Am 2001;83:219–28.
22. Jeng CL, Campbell JT, Tang EY, et al. Tibiotalocalcaneal arthrodesis with bulk femoral head allograft for salvage of large defects in the ankle. Foot Ankle Int 2013;34(9):1256–66.
23. Cuttica DJ, Hyer CF. Femoral head allograft for tibiotalocalcaneal fusion using a cup and cone reamer technique. J Foot Ankle Surg 2011;50(1):126–9.
24. Giaretta S, Micheloni GM, Mazzi M, et al. The "Ball in Basket" Technique for Tibiotalocalcaneal Fusion. Acta Biomed 2020;91(4-S):172–8.
25. Hoang V, Anthony T, Gupta S, et al. Treatment of Severe Ankle and Hindfoot Deformity: Technique Using Femoral Head Allograft for Tibiotalocalcaneal Fusion Using a Cup-and-Cone Reamer. Arthrosc Tech 2021;10(5):e1187–95.
26. Kreulen C, Lian E, Giza E. Technique for Use of Trabecular Metal Spacers in Tibiotalocalcaneal Arthrodesis with Large Bony Defects. Foot Ankle Int 2017;38(1):96–106.
27. Horisberger M, Paul J, Wiewiorski M, et al. Commercially available trabecular metal ankle interpositional spacer for tibiotalocalcaneal arthrodesis secondary to severe bone loss of the ankle. J Foot Ankle Surg 2014;53(3):383–7.

28. Sundet M, Johnsen E, Eikvar KH, et al. Retrograde nailing, trabecular metal implant and use of bone marrow aspirate concentrate after failed ankle joint replacement. Foot Ankle Surg 2021;27(2):123–8.
29. Aubret S, Merlini L, Fessy M, et al. Poor outcomes of fusion with Trabecular Metal implants after failed total ankle replacement: Early results in 11 patients. Orthop Traumatol Surg Res 2018;104(2):231–7.
30. Bejarano-Pineda L, Sharma A, Adams SB, et al. Three-Dimensional Printed Cage in Patients With Tibiotalocalcaneal Arthrodesis Using a Retrograde Intramedullary Nail: Early Outcomes. Foot Ankle Spec 2021;14(5):401–9.
31. Lachman JR, Adams SB. Tibiotalocalcaneal Arthrodesis for Severe Talar Avascular Necrosis. Foot Ankle Clin 2019;24(1):143–61.
32. Sherman AE, Mehta MP, Nayak R, et al. Biologic Augmentation of Tibiotalocalcaneal Arthrodesis with Allogeneic Bone Block Is Associated With High Rates of Fusion. Foot Ankle Int 2022;43(3):353–62.
33. Escudero MI, Poggio D, Alvarez F, et al. Tibiotalocalcaneal arthrodesis with distal tibial allograft for massive bone deficits in the ankle. Foot Ankle Surg 2019;25(3):390–7.
34. Vaughn J, DeFontes KW 3rd, Keyser C, et al. Case Series: Allograft Tibiotalocalcaneal Arthrodesis Utilizing Fresh Talus. Foot Ankle Orthop 2019;4(2). 2473011419834541.
35. Rabiu AR, Mart JS, Reichert ILH, et al. The King's Sliding Hindfoot Osteotomy for the Treatment of Talus Body Defects-Results of a New Technique in Tibiotalocalcaneal Arthrodesis. J Foot Ankle Surg 2021;60(6):1301–7.
36. Hsu AR, Ellington JK, Adams SB Jr. Tibiotalocalcaneal Arthrodesis Using a Nitinol Intramedullary Hindfoot Nail. Foot Ankle Spec 2015;8(5):389–96.
37. Taylor J, Lucas DE, Riley A, et al. Tibiotalocalcaneal Arthrodesis Nails: A Comparison of Nails With and Without Internal Compression. Foot Ankle Int 2016;37(3):294–9.
38. Berson L, McGarvey WC, Clanton TO. Evaluation of compression in intramedullary hindfoot arthrodesis. Foot Ankle Int 2002;23(11):992–5.
39. Niinimäki TT, Klemola TM, Leppilahti JI. Tibiotalocalcaneal arthrodesis with a compressive retrograde intramedullary nail: a report of 34 consecutive patients. Foot Ankle Int 2007;28(4):431–4.
40. Rammelt S, Pyrc J, Agren PH, et al. Tibiotalocalcaneal fusion using the hindfoot arthrodesis nail: a multicenter study. Foot Ankle Int 2013;34(9):1245–55.
41. Perez-Aznar A, Gonzalez-Navarro B, Bello-Tejeda LL, et al. Tibiotalocalcaneal arthrodesis with a retrograde intramedullary nail: a prospective cohort study at a minimum five year follow-up. Int Orthop 2021. https://doi.org/10.1007/s00264-020-04904-3.
42. Richter M, Zech S. Tibiotalocalcaneal arthrodesis with a triple-bend intramedullary nail (A3)-2-year follow-up in 60 patients. Foot Ankle Surg 2016;22(2):131–8.
43. Klaue K, Wichelhaus A, Maik P, et al. The circular arc shaped nail for fixing the tibiotalocalcaneal arthrodesis. After clinical results. Injury 2019;50(Suppl 3):23–31.
44. O'Neill PJ, Parks BG, Walsh R, et al. Biomechanical analysis of screw-augmented intramedullary fixation for tibiotalocalcaneal arthrodesis. Foot Ankle Int 2007;28(7):804–9.
45. Hanson TW, Cracchiolo A 3rd. The use of a 95 degree blade plate and a posterior approach to achieve tibiotalocalcaneal arthrodesis. Foot Ankle Int 2002;23(8):704–10.

46. Ohlson BL, Shatby MW, Parks BG, et al. Periarticular locking plate vs intramedullary nail for tibiotalocalcaneal arthrodesis: a biomechanical investigation. Am J Orthop (Belle Mead Nj) 2011.
47. Kheir E, Borse V, Bryant H, et al. The use of the 4.5 mm 90° titanium cannulated LC-angled blade plate in tibiotalocalcaneal and complex ankle arthrodesis. Foot Ankle Surg 2015;21(4):240–4.
48. Chodos MD, Parks BG, Schon LC, et al. Blade plate compared with locking plate for tibiotalocalcaneal arthrodesis: a cadaver study. Foot Ankle Int 2008;29(2):219–24.
49. Yao Y, Mo Z, Wu G, et al. A personalized 3D-printed plate for tibiotalocalcaneal arthrodesis: Design, fabrication, biomechanical evaluation and postoperative assessment. Comput Biol Med 2021;133:104368.
50. Alfahd U, Roth SE, Stephen D, et al. Biomechanical comparison of intramedullary nail and blade plate fixation for tibiotalocalcaneal arthrodesis. J Orthop Trauma 2005;19(10):703–8.
51. Froelich J, Idusuyi OB, Clark D, et al. Torsional stiffness of an intramedullary nail versus blade plate fixation for tibiotalocalcaneal arthrodesis: a biomechanical study. J Surg Orthop Adv 2010;19(2):109–13.
52. Hamid KS, Glisson RR, Morash JG, et al. Simultaneous Intraoperative Measurement of Cadaver Ankle and Subtalar Joint Compression During Arthrodesis with Intramedullary Nail, Screws, and Tibiotalocalcaneal Plate. Foot Ankle Int 2018;39(9):1128–32.
53. Chiodo CP, Acevedo JI, Sammarco VJ, et al. Intramedullary rod fixation compared with blade-plate-and-screw fixation for tibiotalocalcaneal arthrodesis: a biomechanical investigation. J Bone Joint Surg Am 2003;85(12):2425–8.
54. Gutteck N, Schilde S, Reichel M, et al. Posterolateral plate fixation with Pantalarlock® is more stable than nail fixation in tibiotalocalcaneal arthrodesis in a biomechanical cadaver study. Foot Ankle Surg 2020;26(3):328–33.
55. Santangelo JR, Glisson RR, Garras DN, et al. Tibiotalocalcaneal arthrodesis: a biomechanical comparision of multiplanar external fixation with intramedullary fixation. Foot Ankle Int 2008;29(9):936–41.
56. Richman J, Cota A, Weinfeld S. Intramedullary Nailing and External Ring Fixation for Tibiotalocalcaneal Arthrodesis in Charcot Arthropathy. Foot Ankle Int 2017;38(2):149–52.
57. Paul J, Barg A, Horisberger M, et al. Ankle salvage surgery with autologous circular pillar fibula augmentation and intramedullary hindfoot nail. J Foot Ankle Surg 2014;53(5):601–5.
58. Bernasconi A, Patel S, Malhotra K, et al. Salvage Tibiotalocalcaneal Arthrodesis Augmented With Fibular Columns and Iliac Crest Autograft: A Technical Note. Foot Ankle Spec 2021;14(1):79–88.
59. Shah AB, Jones C, Elattar O, et al. Tibiotalocalcaneal Arthrodesis With Intramedullary Fibular Strut Graft With Adjuvant Hardware Fixation. J Foot Ankle Surg 2017;56(3):692–6.
60. Roukis TS, Kang RB. Vascularized Pedicled Fibula Onlay Bone Graft Augmentation for Complicated Tibiotalocalcaneal Arthrodesis with Retrograde Intramedullary Nail Fixation: A Case Series. J Foot Ankle Surg 2016;55(4):857–67.
61. Watanabe K, Teramoto A, Kobayashi T, et al. Tibiotalocalcaneal Arthrodesis Using a Soft-tissue-Preserved Fibular Graft for Treatment of Large Bone Defects in the Ankle. Foot Ankle Int 2017;38(6):671–6.

62. Mulhern JL, Protzman NM, Levene MJ, et al. Is Subtalar Joint Cartilage Resection Necessary for Tibiotalocalcaneal Arthrodesis via Intramedullary Nail? A Multicenter Evaluation. J Foot Ankle Surg 2016;55(3):572–7.

63. Dujela M, Hyer CF, Berlet GC. Rate of Subtalar Joint Arthrodesis After Retrograde Tibiotalocalcaneal Arthrodesis with Intramedullary Nail Fixation: Evaluation of the RAIN Database. Foot Ankle Spec 2018;11(5):410–5.

64. Yoshimoto K, Fukushi JI, Tsushima H, et al. Does Preparation of the Subtalar Joint for Primary Union Affect Clinical Outcome in Patients Undergoing Intramedullary Nail for Rheumatoid Arthritis of the Hindfoot and Ankle? J Foot Ankle Surg 2020; 59(5):984–7.

65. Sealey RJ, Myerson MS, Molloy A, et al. Sagittal plane motion of the hindfoot following ankle arthrodesis: a prospective analysis. Foot Ankle Int 2009;30(3): 187–96.

66. Chopra S, Crevoisier X. Bilateral gait asymmetry associated with tibiotalocalcaneal arthrodesis versus ankle arthrodesis. Foot Ankle Surg 2020. S1268-7731(20)30265-4.

67. Burns PR, Dunse A. Tibiotalocalcaneal Arthrodesis for Foot and Ankle Deformities. Clin Podiatr Med Surg 2017;34(3):357–80.

68. Patel S, Baker L, Perez J, et al. Risk factors for nonunion following tibiotalocalcaneal arthrodesis: A systematic review and meta-analysis. Foot Ankle Surg 2021. S1268-7731(21)00036-9.

69. Levinson J, Reissig J, Schaheen E, et al. Complications and Radiographic Outcomes After Tibiotalocalcaneal Fusion with a Retrograde Intramedullary Nail. Foot Ankle Spec 2020. 1938640020950153.

70. Pitts C, Alexander B, Washington J, et al. Factors affecting the outcomes of tibiotalocalcaneal fusion. Bone Joint J 2020;102-B(3):345–51.

71. Cooper PS. Complications of ankle and tibiotalocalcaneal arthrodesis. Clin Orthop Relat Res 2001;391:33–44.

72. Fuchs S, Sandmann C, Skwara A, et al. Quality of life 20 years after arthrodesis of the ankle a study of adjacent joints. J Bone Joint Surg Br 2003;85:994–8.

73. Mehta MP, Mehta MP, Sherman AE, et al. Evaluating Prospective Patient-Reported Pain and Function Outcomes After Ankle and Hindfoot Arthrodesis. Foot Ankle Orthop 2021;6(4). 24730114211040740.

74. Mencière ML, Ferraz L, Mertl P, et al. Arthroscopic tibiotalocalcaneal arthrodesis in neurological pathologies: outcomes after at least one year of follow up. Acta Orthop Belg 2016;82(1):106–11.

75. Franceschi F, Franceschetti E, Torre G, et al. Tibiotalocalcaneal arthrodesis using an intramedullary nail: a systematic review. Knee Surg Sports Traumatol Arthrosc 2016;24(4):1316–25.

76. Powers NS, Brandao RA, St John JM, et al. Outcomes and Management of Infected Intramedullary Nails After Tibiotalocalcaneal Arthrodesis in Limb Salvage: A Retrospective Case Series. J Foot Ankle Surg 2020;59(2):431–5.

77. Powers NS, Leatham PR, Persky JD, et al. Outcomes of Tibiotalocalcaneal Arthrodesis with a Femoral Nail. J Am Podiatr Med Assoc 2021;111(3):4. https://doi.org/10.7547/19-151.

78. Rogero R, Tsai J, Fuchs D, et al. Midterm Results of Radiographic and Functional Outcomes After Tibiotalocalcaneal Arthrodesis With Bulk Femoral Head Allograft. Foot Ankle Spec 2020;13(4):315–23.

79. Stołtny T, Dugiełło B, Pasek J, et al. Tibiotalocalcaneal Arthrodesis in Osteoarthritis Deformation of Ankle and Subtalar Joint: Evaluation of Treatment Results. J Foot Ankle Surg 2022;61(1):205–11.

80. Jehan S, Shakeel M, Bing AJ, et al. The success of tibiotalocalcaneal arthrodesis with intramedullary nailing–a systematic review of the literature. Acta Orthop Belg 2011;77(5):644–51.
81. Tirrell AR, Kim KG, Rashid W, et al. Patient-reported Outcome Measures following Traumatic Lower Extremity Amputation: A Systematic Review and Meta-analysis. Plast Reconstr Surg Glob Open 2021;9(11):e3920.

Ankle Arthrodesis in Crippled Cases

Norman Espinosa, MD

KEYWORDS

• Arthrodesis • Algorithm • Complex • Deformities • Plan

KEY POINTS

• Complex ankle deformities can be difficult to treat.
• Complex ankle deformities may need an interdisciplinary approach.
• Complex deformities may need multiple steps in order to achieve the goal.
• The most efficient way to approach the problem: the least necessary to get the best result.
• There is no standard ankle pathology and no standard treatment available: everything remains custom-made.

INTRODUCTION

Although joint preserving surgery has gained a lot of attention in the treatment ankle disorders, there still remain deformities, which will require arthrodesis to solve the problem.[1–4] Those deformities include pathologies, which are not amenable to osteotomies, soft-tissue reconstruction, and arthroplasties alone. In addition, any of those cases bear an inherently present and increased risk for potential complications.

Precise preparation before embarking on such kind of interventions is mandatory and frequently multidisciplinary. When fusing the ankle joint it will transfer forces to the adjacent ones, leading to compensatory movement and more or less pronounced, mechanical overload.[5] This effect will certainly result in secondary degeneration of the adjacent joints. When additional fusions are attempted (besides the ankle joint), this effect gets accelerated.

Thus, foot and ankle surgeons should follow the most efficient way to correct the deformity through arthrodesis: the least necessary to achieve the greatest correction and success.

The current article tries to outline an algorithm of how to approach those deformities and to offer some thoughts regarding treatment.

Institute for Foot and Ankle Reconstruction, FussInstitut Zurich, Beethovenstrasse 3, Zurich 8002, Switzerland
E-mail address: espinosa@fussinstitut.ch

Foot Ankle Clin N Am 27 (2022) 867–881
https://doi.org/10.1016/j.fcl.2022.07.004
1083-7515/22/© 2022 Elsevier Inc. All rights reserved.

foot.theclinics.com

It is absolutely important to realize that no standard ankle pathology or treatment exists and thus an individual selection of techniques and surgical approaches is required.

In conclusion, surgeons who will have to deal with those kinds of deformities should be equipped with the full foot and ankle armamentarium available; this includes not only the surgical techniques but also the clinical assessment and imaging technologies.

WHAT KIND OF DEFORMITY IS PRESENT?

This is the principal question. It is based on the clinical and radiographic examination.
The main characteristics of a deformity are as follows:

- Single deformity, that is, at a single spot
- Multiple deformities, that is, at multiple spots
- Flexible
- Rigid
- Combination of rigid and flexible deformities

Clinical Assessment

The clinical assessment involves inspection, palpation, and functional testing. A proper, clinical examination elicits not only the type of deformity but also its shapeable properties, that is, whether it is flexible or rigid.

The current article does not go into all details of physical examination and focuses on specific aspects of the topic discussed herein.

Manual testing allows the identification of the amount of rigidity or flexibility. It ensures the possibility to examine whether a deformity can passively be reduced into neutral or not.

As a specific entity, it is also necessary to distinguish between a forefoot-driven hindfoot varus and forefoot-driven hindfoot valgus deformity.[6,7] The latter is not well known. However, with regard to the kinematic chain of the foot and ankle it obviously must exist.

During testing the result will be classified as a hypermobile first ray, which can take place everywhere in the medial column, starting at the first tarsometatarsal joint (TMT-I-joint) and running through the naviculocuneiform or talonavicular joint.[8-11] In some patients even the entire medial column can be unstable, complicating the final surgical strategy. To assess a forefoot-driven hindfoot valgus the author does not only refer to the manual testing but uses the so-called reversed Coleman-block test.[12]

When examining a forefoot-driven hindfoot varus deformity the "Coleman-block" test helps to identify whether the hindfoot varus is flexible or not.[12] In addition to the Coleman-block test, any hyperactivity of the peroneus longus should be verified.[7]

In case of highly rigid deformities, the clinical assessment will reach to a limit where no reduction can be achieved. Under such circumstances imaging techniques can serve a lot and help to depict the deformity as well as its pitfalls for the surgical planning.

Clinical assessment of the arterial pulses (Aa. popliteal, dorsalis pedis, and tibialis posterior) is absolutely necessary. If there is any doubt of vascular impairment, an angiological (including angiography) examination should be ordered.

Radiographic Assessment

In general, the apex of deformity can be assessed by using a conventional radiograph and identifying the center of rotation of angulation (ie, CORA).

The author always uses 5 conventional radiographic views under weight-bearing conditions:

- Anteroposterior view of the ankle
- Long-axial view of the hindfoot
- Lateral view of the foot
- Dorsoplantar view of the foot
- Oblique view of the foot

Other, more sophisticated, imaging techniques, for example, MRI, computed tomography (CT), and single-photon emission computerized tomography-CT, help to assess the presence of osteoarthritis and its expansion, the integrity of the soft tissues (ie, tendons, ligaments, cartilage, and so forth), and the status of perfusion.[13]

More recently, foot and ankle surgeons have paid much attention to the weight-bearing CT scans (WBCT scans).[14] A WBCT scan allows to examine a deformity in its 3 dimensions. Thus, it has become accepted as a very important tool to investigate the nature of complex deformities, for example, progressive collapsing foot deformities.[15]

WHAT KIND OF STRUCTURAL PROBLEMS SHOULD BE LOOKED AT?

Complex deformities can involve various structures and therefore complicate surgical planning and performance.

It might be of value to look at the specific problems that may be associated with complex deformities before embarking on treatment strategies.

The author attempts to provide an overview, which starts from the superficial until reaching to the core of the foot and ankle:

- Skin and approaches
- Vascular supply
- Muscle contractures
- Capsular stiffness
- Bones
- Techniques

Skin and Approaches

The skin plays an elementary role during selection of the surgical approach. The optimal approach is direct and should not harm important structures, which are not involved in the pathology. One of the most important aspects is that wound closure could be achieved at the end of a procedure.

Surgeons need to take into consideration that whenever a correction will be performed at the foot and ankle, the skin incision should be chosen in a manner that allows proper wound healing. For example, in a severe hindfoot valgus, where a diple arthrodesis is planned together with an ankle fusion (pantalar fusion), a medial skin incision alone is far better than a combination of a lateral and medial incision.[16–18] The latter increases the risk of spreading wound edges after correction of the valgus into neutral, preventing proper closure.

Besides this, skin incisions should be performed at places where the angiosomes are respected the most[19,20]; this avoids further wound healing problems.

Patients who have already been treated surgically may have scars, which result in precarious skin conditions. In those cases, an alternative approach should be thought over. If not possible, a surgeon should be prepared to involve a temporary wound vacuum dressing and plastic surgeon to help cover the skin.

Ankle joint: the author prefers, whenever possible, an anterior approach to the ankle. The primary goal is to preserve the anatomy and geometry of the hindfoot at best; this may be important in patients in whom a total ankle replacement will be considered in the future.

However, if not feasible or when the deformity dictates another option, a lateral approach or even posterior approach need to be considered.

In cases where the tibia should be addressed and the fibula is part of the deformity (while requiring correction), a separate lateral incision is almost always needed.

Subtalar joint: when there is not much deformity present, a lateral approach might be sufficient. However, in patients who will need any type of distraction at the subtalar joint (by implantation of a bone graft), the posterior approach through a longitudinal skin incision over the Achilles tendon should be preferred, which avoids the risk of inability to close the skin.

Lisfranc joint: a simple TMT-I fusion can be done through a small dorsomedial or medial incision over the joint. When addressing the first ray and lateral rays together, a 2-incision technique is required. The minimal distance between the incisions averages at least 2 finger widths.[21]

Vascular Supply

Proper perfusion provides a sound base for healing. The more complex a deformity is, the greater the risk for potential vascular problems. In patients suffering from deformities after trauma, it is mandatory to check whether a proper vascular supply is present or not. In those cases, vascular studies should be considered in order to rule out any vascular impairment.

Muscle Contractures

Some deformities include quite tight contractures of the musculature. Those might be the result of a long-standing atrophy and fatty infiltration of the muscle tissue. The origin of muscle contracture can have various causes: traumatic disruption of the muscle tissue, long-standing immobilization, neurologic disorders/lesions and idiopathic causes.[22–24]

With regard to the foot and ankle, the triceps surae is the most important muscle unit, which can be affected by contracture. As a result, the foot will turn into an equinus position. In order to correct the equinus, an Achilles tendon lengthening will be necessary, which can be done percutaneously by 3 stab incisions (analogous to the method described by Hoke) or open depending on the magnitude of deformity.[25–28]

The author prefers a percutaneous Achilles tendon lengthening in light-to-moderate equinus deformities (up to 10°). For all other equinus deformities a z-shaped lengthening is performed.

Capsular Stiffness

Capsular stiffness is a condition, which could impair proper reduction of the bones during fusion. To the author's opinion, it is necessary to think about those capsular stiffnesses because they influence the surgical plan.

For example, in patients with a severe equinocavovarus deformity, the medial talonavicular joint capsule, including the deltoid and spring ligament, is quite frequently found stiff and contract. In order to derotate the Chopart joint, it is mandatory to perform a capsulotomy, that is, a full release.

Sometimes an equinus malposition of the hindfoot is primarily caused by a stiffness or fibrosis of the posterior ankle ± subtalar joint capsule. In such cases the posterior compartment of the hindfoot will need a complete release to allow proper reduction of the bones.

Bones

Finally, the bones are the anatomical structures that need to be reduced and fused. Before embarking on surgery, it is important to figure out how the bones are altered in their anatomical structure:

- Bones are normal in shape
- Bones are normal in shape but misaligned
- Bones are abnormally shaped
- Bones are abnormally shaped and associated with misalignment
- Bones have already been fused by a surgeon but misaligned
- Bones present with partial or complete avascular necrosis

In patients with clubfeet or severe hindfoot cavovarus deformity misshaped bones are frequently found.[29] Those bony alterations pose significant problems in order to achieve an anatomical restoration of the foot and ankle. Even in the context of ankle fusion those alterations of anatomical shape and structure can require major corrections, which increase the risk for complications.

Coalitions of bones or bones that have been fused in a previous surgery may need a surgical separation before starting with the final procedure.

In patients who present with partial or complete avascular necrosis, the risk for a nonunion is increased. Thus, improved vascularization should be provided, which may need a vascularized bone graft.

Techniques

A surgeon who will treat challenging deformities needs to be familiar with all aspects of the foot and ankle armamentarium:

- Ankle fusion
  - Implants
    - Anterior plate
    - Posterior plate
    - Crossed-screws
    - Lateral plate
    - Nailing systems
  - Bone grafts
    - Allograft
    - Autograft
    - Vascularized graft
  - Osteotomies
    - Bone-wedge/bone removal
    - Opening-wedge technique
    - Dome osteotomies
- Subtalar fusion
  - Implants
    - Screws
  - Distraction arthrodesis using a bone graft
    - Allograft

- Autograft
- Vascularized graft
  - Bone separation
    - Coalitions
  - Lateral bone resection
- Tibiotalocalcaneal fusion
  - Same as listed under sections Ankle Fusion and Subtalar Fusion
- Diple arthrodesis
  - Implants
    - Screws only
    - Screws and plates
  - Interposition of bone graft
    - Allograft
    - Autograft
    - Vascularized bone graft
- Lisfranc arthrodesis
  - Implants
    - Screws only
    - Screws and plates
    - Plates only
  - Interposition of bone graft
    - Allograft
    - Autograft
    - Vascularized bone graft
- Atypical fusions (eg, fusion of ankle joint + calcaneocuboid joint)
  - Implants
    - Screws and plates
  - Interposition of bone graft
    - Allograft
    - Autograft
    - Vascularized bone graft

HOW TO MANAGE CHALLENGING DEFORMITIES WITH ARTHRODESIS OF THE ANKLE

The previous paragraphs served to explain the rational of thinking regarding challenging deformities and their treatment. The author tried to provide a certain algorithm of how to approach those patients. It is clear that sometimes not only the ankle joint but also other joints require fusion. Although the latter is not the primary focus of the current article, the author thinks that this is important to look at.

In the following paragraphs the author guides the reader through some specific cases of challenging deformities. The way of treatment follows the algorithm previously presented in this article. As mentioned, those examples are all unique: no standard patient and no standard treatment exists. Of course, we will not be able to look at all possible cases, but the current examples would like to show how to approach patients with difficult and complex deformities.

Case Example

This is the case of a 48-year-old female patient who has sustained a severe right talar fracture due to a frontal collision in motor vehicle accident (**Fig. 1**). The patient has initially been treated for her polytrauma (ISS17); this took place in a University Center.

The talar body was smashed into various pieces with a predominant destruction of the medial area (**Fig. 2**). The talar body was addressed by open reduction and internal reduction through a medial malleolar osteotomy (**Fig. 3**).

Almost one year after the talar reconstruction the patient was referred to the author's clinic for further evaluation. At that time the patient reported significant pain and that other surgeons proposed to perform a tibiocalcaneal arthrodesis of the hindfoot by means of an intramedullary nail.

The patient was quite well aware of the fact that a tibiocalcaneal arthrodesis would shorten the leg and sacrifice the subtalar joint. Thus, the patient sought a second opinion. The main question of the patient was whether a hindfoot reconstruction could be done in order to preserve the subtalar joint while maintaining proper length of the leg.

At initial presentation the patient suffered from severe pain and inability to walk.

Clinical assessment showed a remarkable equinus position of the hindfoot and varus malalignment. Because of the equinus malposition the patient started to compensate this deformity through a hyperextension in the right knee joint.

The ankle joint was quite tender to palpation, whereas the subtalar joint did not reveal any pain. The Chopart and Lisfranc joints were intact. Neither neurological nor vascular impairment (ie, intact and well-perfused Aa. dorsalis pedis and tibialis posterior) was found.

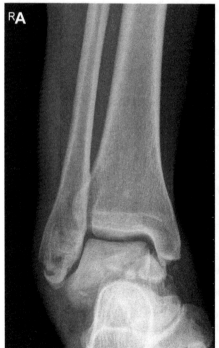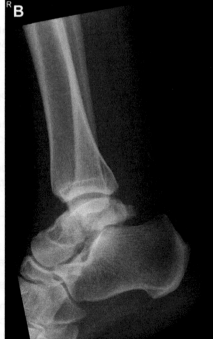

Fig. 1. (*A*) Depicted is the anteroposterior view of the right ankle. Note the subtalar dislocation and irregularities in the body of talus itself. In addition, the tip of the fibula is broken. (*B*) Lateral view of the same patient. The talar body fracture has led to a flattening of the body structure. Incongruent subtalar joint.

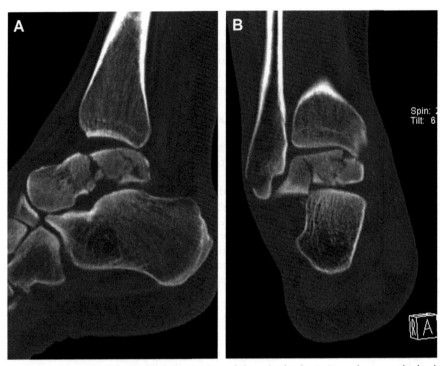

Fig. 2. (*A*) CT scan with sagittal reconstruction of the talar body. As it can be seen, the body shows a comminuted fracture type. (*B*) Coronal reconstruction of the talus on CT. The talus is widened in the mediolateral extension. Please note the predominant involvement of the medial talar body.

Radiographic assessment revealed a progressive necrosis of the talar body (**Figs. 4 and 5**).

In order to get a better appreciation of the hindfoot a CT scan has been performed. The CT scan showed the necrotic talar body with involvement of the subtalar joint (**Fig. 6**).

Therefore, the final diagnosis was *malunion and severe osteoarthritis of right ankle and subtalar joint due to osteonecrosis of the talus.*

Treatment Plan

1. Goal:

Reconstruction of the talus, as anatomic as possible to allow an adequate fusion of the ankle joint, while preserving the subtalar joint.

2. Important and specific points in this case:

The perfusion of the right talar bone is nonexistent. Thus, vascularity needs to be brought to the talar bone, which can be achieved by transfer of a vascularized bone graft of the medial femoral condyle. This surgery needs a plastic surgeon and an angiography of the entire lower leg. The transferred autograft should not be compressed by or fixed through an implant. The goal here is to preserve a proper perfusion of the vascularized bone graft.

To reconstruct the talar body, a separate bone graft is needed.

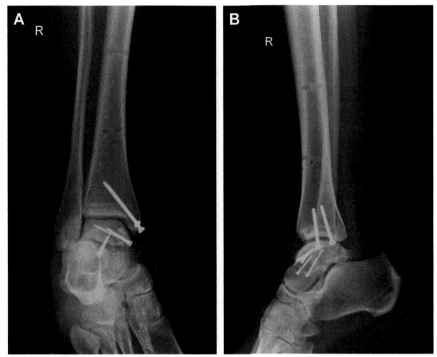

Fig. 3. (*A*) Anteroposterior view of the ankle after open reduction and internal fixation through a medial malleolar osteotomy. (*B*) Lateral view of the same foot. The talus could be reconstructed in a nice way. The subtalar joint is anatomically reduced.

3. Approach:

An anterior approach to ankle allows the direct visualization of the entire talar bone. The reconstruction of the talar body can be done through this approach, whereas the connection of the vascularized medial femoral condyle autograft can be connected to the A. dorsalis pedis.

4. Implants:

An autologous or allogenic bone graft.

Vascularized medial femoral condyle allograft, which will be placed anterior onto the talar dome.

An anterior plate offers best fixation, while allowing the placement of the vascularized bone graft without compression.

5. Achilles tendon lengthening:

This needs to be done because the foot is positioned in equinus. The author used a 3-incision technique.

Surgery

The woman was operated on her right hindfoot after meticulous planning of the surgery. Through an anterior approach the talar body could be reached. The posterior cartilage of the talar dome was still viable. In the center a massive defect zone could be found. As a primary technique the dead bone has been removed carefully by means

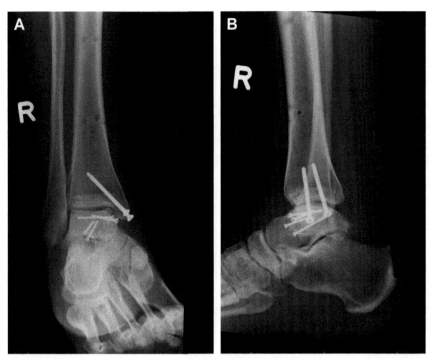

Fig. 4. (*A*) Postoperative anteroposterior view of the right ankle. This is 3 months after surgery. The talar dome reveals certain irregularities on the medial side. (*B*) First signs of a slight collapse of the talar body can be seen. On top of the talus the bone has become sclerotic (Hawkins sign).

of a curette and osteotome. The subtalar joint could not be seen because the cartilage worked as a local sealing structure. Thus, allogenic bone could be inserted until the entire core of the talar body was filled with it. Under fluoroscopic control the result of the reconstruction could be checked. The primary issue with this technique is penetration of the subtalar joint and dissemination of bone graft within the subtalar joint; this was not the case in this specific patient.

The vascularized medial femoral bone graft was then connected onto the A. dorsalis pedis and laid directly in front of the ankle joint. The anterior, solid plate was then first fixed on the talar head and then secured onto the tibia. During this step, it was absolutely important the vascularized bone graft was kept secure without any pressure exerted by the implant.

After the surgery the perfusion of the vascularized bone graft was regularly checked by means of a Doppler ultrasound.

Six weeks postoperatively the patient presented with a clinically well oriented right hindfoot and was very satisfied with the result (**Fig. 7**). The pain has gone as he reported.

Three months postoperatively the patient still presented with a well-aligned hindfoot and a fusion of the ankle joint (**Fig. 8**). Free ambulation has been commenced.

Four years after this surgery, the patient is still very satisfied with the result. She is able to walk without pain in the ankle joint. Some pain in the subtalar joint has started to begin. However, currently the patient does not wish to continue with a further treatment because the discomfort is minimal.

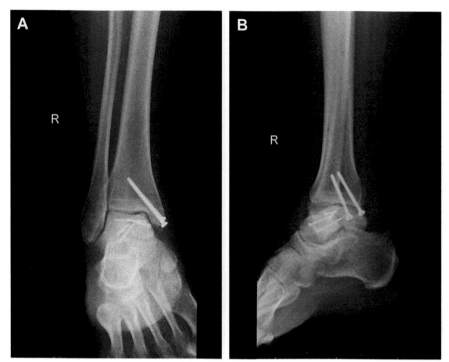

Fig. 5. (A) The white appearance of the talar body is enhanced. Osteonecrosis is now manifest. (B) On the lateral view of the foot the correction, that is, reconstruction got lost. The bone starts to crack into fragments.

WHAT WE SHOULD LEARN

Challenging ankle deformities are difficult to treat. They require a thorough preparation and surgeons need to accept that in some specific cases corrections cannot be done by a single intervention alone because the risks of complications would outweigh the benefits for the patient.

In those cases, a multistep strategy needs to be considered. Besides this, some patients in whom challenging deformities are found may need a multidisciplinary approach to their pathologies. At least in the preoperative setting, adequate planning becomes the corner stone of management.

Each of those cases is unique. No standard pathology exists. Therefore, there is also no standardized treatment strategy available; this complicates the ways to solve the problems properly.

A thorough knowledge in foot and ankle surgery and wide experience in clinical assessment of the patients is mandatory to cope with all challenging deformities. In addition, the surgeon should be familiar with the entire surgical armamentarium. As already mentioned, it is not sufficient to have a plan A. No: a surgeon needs also to have a plan B and C, and so forth. This means that patients should also be aware of this fact.

However, if an adequate planning can be performed the execution of the surgical intervention becomes more secure associated with a higher probability of success.

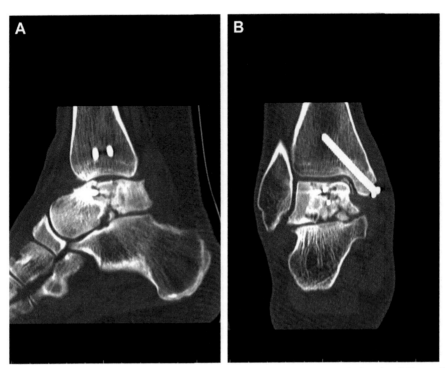

Fig. 6. (*A*) On CT scan the loss of reduction, the necrotic process, and also the failure of consolidation can be seen. It involves the subtalar joint too. (*B*) In the coronal view the talar bone does not show any sign of union.

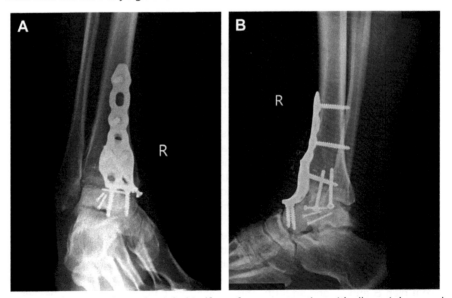

Fig. 7. (*A*) This image shows the right hindfoot after reconstruction with allogenic bone and application of a vascularized medial femoral condyle autograft on the front of the ankle. Fixation could be achieved by means of an anterior plate. (*B*) On the lateral view of the hindfoot the reconstruction of the talar body can very well be appreciated. The subtalar joint has also been corrected.

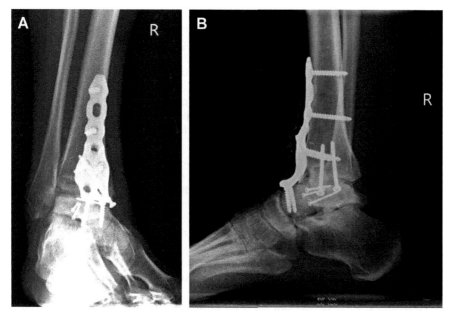

Fig. 8. (*A*) The anteroposterior view of the ankle joint reveals the solid union 6 months post-operatively. No failure of the implant can be seen. (*B*) On the lateral view of the ankle joint the position of the ankle is well and the subtalar joint stable.

CLINICS CARE POINTS

- Complex and challenging deformities at the ankle are high demanding cases.
- Surgeons who deal with those deformities need to be familiar with all techniques and should be aware of their individual, complex character.
- Meticulous planning and careful execution of the surgery is mandatory to achieve a satisfying outcome for the patient.
- Sometimes multiple steps within well-defined time intervals between the interventions are necessary to achieve a complete reconstruction of the foot and ankle.

REFERENCES

1. Hintermann B, et al. The use of supramalleolar osteotomies in posttraumatic deformity and arthritis of the ankle. JBJS Essent Surg Tech 2017;7(4):e29.
2. Rammelt S, Zwipp H. [Joint-preserving correction of Chopart joint malunions]. Unfallchirurg 2014;117(9):785–90.
3. Rammelt S, Marti RK, Zwipp H. [Joint-preserving osteotomy of malunited ankle and pilon fractures]. Unfallchirurg 2013;116(9):789–96.
4. Hintermann B, Knupp M, Barg A. Joint-preserving surgery of asymmetric ankle osteoarthritis with peritalar instability. Foot Ankle Clin 2013;18(3):503–16.

5. Coester LM, et al. Long-term results following ankle arthrodesis for post-traumatic arthritis. J Bone Joint Surg Am 2001;83(2):219–28.
6. Espinosa N, Klammer G. The failed deltoid ligament in the valgus misaligned ankle-how to treat? Foot Ankle Clin 2021;26(2):391–405.
7. Klammer G, Benninger E, Espinosa N. The varus ankle and instability. Foot Ankle Clin 2012;17(1):57–82.
8. Cowie S, et al. Hypermobility of the first ray in patients with planovalgus feet and tarsometatarsal osteoarthritis. Foot Ankle Surg 2012;18(4):237–40.
9. Myerson MS, Badekas A. Hypermobility of the first ray. Foot Ankle Clin 2000;5(3): 469–84.
10. Prieskorn DW, Mann RA, Fritz G. Radiographic assessment of the second metatarsal: measure of first ray hypermobility. Foot Ankle Int 1996;17(6):331–3.
11. Klaue K, Hansen ST, Masquelet AC. Clinical, quantitative assessment of first tarsometatarsal mobility in the sagittal plane and its relation to hallux valgus deformity. Foot Ankle Int 1994;15(1):9–13.
12. Wood EV, Syed A, Geary NP. Clinical tip: the reverse coleman block test radiograph. Foot Ankle Int 2009;30(7):708–10.
13. Zanetti M, Saupe N, Espinosa N. Postoperative MR imaging of the foot and ankle: tendon repair, ligament repair, and Morton's neuroma resection. Semin Musculoskelet Radiol 2010;14(3):357–64.
14. Hirschmann A, et al. Upright cone CT of the hindfoot: comparison of the non-weight-bearing with the upright weight-bearing position. Eur Radiol 2014;24(3): 553–8.
15. de Cesar Netto C, et al. Consensus for the use of weightbearing CT in the assessment of progressive collapsing foot deformity. Foot Ankle Int 2020;41(10): 1277–82.
16. So E, et al. Medial Double Arthrodesis: Technique Guide and Tips. J Foot Ankle Surg 2018;57(2):364–9.
17. Knupp M, et al. Medial approach to the subtalar joint: anatomy, indications, technique tips. Foot Ankle Clin 2015;20(2):311–8.
18. Weinraub GM, et al. Isolated medial incisional approach to subtalar and talonavicular arthrodesis. J Foot Ankle Surg 2010;49(4):326–30.
19. Ferraresi R, et al. Foot angiosomes: instructions for use. Int J Low Extrem Wounds 2020;19(4):293–304.
20. Settembre N, et al. Competing risk analysis of the impact of pedal arch status and angiosome-targeted revascularization in chronic limb-threatening ischemia. Ann Vasc Surg 2020;68:384–90.
21. Uppal HS. Open reduction internal fixation of the lisfranc complex. J Orthop Trauma 2018;32(Suppl 1):S42–3.
22. Ruzbarsky JJ, Scher D, Dodwell E. Toe walking: causes, epidemiology, assessment, and treatment. Curr Opin Pediatr 2016;28(1):40–6.
23. Cychosz CC, et al. Gastrocnemius recession for foot and ankle conditions in adults: Evidence-based recommendations. Foot Ankle Surg 2015;21(2):77–85.
24. Baumann JU. [Treatment of pediatric spastic foot deformities]. Orthopade 1986; 15(3):191–8.
25. Grant AD, Feldman R, Lehman WB. Equinus deformity in cerebral palsy: a retrospective analysis of treatment and function in 39 cases. J Pediatr Orthop 1985; 5(6):678–81.
26. Fadel M, Kandil MF. Management of neglected clubfoot in children using Ilizarov external fixator and minimal invasive surgery, Sub-Saharan Africa experience. Int Orthop 2022;46(1):125–32.

27. Hegewald KW, et al. Minimally invasive approach to achilles tendon pathology. J Foot Ankle Surg 2016;55(1):166–8.
28. Krupinski M, Borowski A, Synder M. Long Term follow-up of subcutaneous achilles tendon lengthening in the treatment of spastic equinus foot in patients with cerebral palsy. Ortop Traumatol Rehabil 2015;17(2):155–61.
29. van der Steen MC, et al. Quantifying joint stiffness in clubfoot patients. Clin Biomech (Bristol, Avon) 2018;60:185–90.

Pantalar Arthrodesis

Sagar Chawla, MD, MPH[a],*, Michael Brage, MD[b]

KEYWORDS

- Pantalar arthrodesis • Pantalar fusion • Pantalar arthritis

KEY POINTS

- Pantalar arthrodesis is a surgical option to provide a stable base for weightbearing in patients with severe deformity, bone loss, and with low physical demand.
- There are several approaches and fixation strategies that result in successful clinical union and should be chosen to match the clinical situation.
- Modern techniques of subtalar, tibiotalar, and transtarsal joint arthrodesis result in high rates of osseous union, pain relief, and patient satisfaction.

INTRODUCTION

A pantalar arthrodesis is triple arthrodesis combined with tibiotalar arthrodesis. A triple arthrodesis is comprised of subtalar, talonavicular, and calcaneocuboid joints arthrodesis. The goal of the procedure is to obtain a correction of deformity and achieve a plantigrade, functional, painless, stable, weightbearing foot that can be used to ambulate. This is done by creating an osseous continuity across the ankle, subtalar, and talonavicular, and calcaneocuboid joints.

The principal indication for pantalar arthrodesis is degenerative or inflammatory arthritis, posterior tibial tendon deficiency with resultant degenerative joint disease, posttraumatic osteoarthritis,[1] deformity[2,3] (either developmental or acquired including ball and socket ankle), sequelae of osteomyelitis[4] (including tuberculosis of the foot and ankle), flaccid paralysis from neuromuscular conditions (poliomyelitis), cerebral palsy, and Charcot joint.

NATURE OF DIAGNOSIS

Historically the primary indication for arthrodesis of the hindfoot was flaccid paralysis caused by neuromuscular conditions, in particular poliomyelitis.[5–8] Polio caused significant morbidity in the first half of the twentieth century. Orthoses used to restore stability to flail lower extremities were heavy, cumbersome, and uncomfortable.[9] Procedures were developed to make the paralytic limb into a useful, plantigrade

[a] Department of Orthopaedics and Sports Medicine, University of Washington, Seattle, WA, USA; [b] Department of Orthopaedics and Sports Medicine, University of Washington, Ninth & Jefferson Building, 908 Jefferson Street, Seattle, WA 98104, USA
* Corresponding author. 4425 Sharon Road, Apartment MPH22, Charlotte, NC 28211.
E-mail address: sagarschawla@gmail.com
Twitter: @sagarschawla (S.C.)

Foot Ankle Clin N Am 27 (2022) 883–895
https://doi.org/10.1016/j.fcl.2022.08.002
1083-7515/22/© 2022 Elsevier Inc. All rights reserved.

foot.theclinics.com

appendage suitable for weightbearing. Early attempts at soft tissue manipulation failed because of tissue attenuation and insufficient motor strength after tendon transfer in the paralytic extremity. Extra-articular bone block procedures were ineffective because of subsequent increase in deformity at adjacent joints and resorption of the bone block.[6,10-12] Talectomy for paralytic feet resulted in significant deformity and subsequently was abandoned.

Hindfoot and ankle arthrodesis were effective at providing stability for the paralytic extremity and were used extensively for treatment of poliomyelitis. Early techniques included talectomy, wide skin exposures, and concomitant tenotomies resulting in complications, with high incidence of postoperative osteonecrosis, flap ischemia and wound healing issues, and stiffness distal to the fusion.[8,13-15] Internal fixation was initially done using boiled cadaver allograft struts, ivory, fibular autograft, or sutures.[11] Progress in techniques resulted in prolonged periods of immobilization and restricted weightbearing. Nonunion was considered successful if outcome was a painless limb that was stable enough for ambulation without bracing.

Modern techniques were pioneered for ankle and foot fusion for complex deformities associated with polio and neuromuscular disease.[5,7,12,16-18] *American Academy of Orthopaedic Surgeons* recommendation in the 1920s was that tendon transfer alone is inadequate. Outcomes studies were done in the 1950s looking at fusion rates, satisfaction, and effect of arthrodesis on the surrounding joints of the foot. The evolution of technique led to a widening of indications, including posttraumatic arthritis, Charcot joint, osteonecrosis, clubfoot deformities, deformities subsequent to posterior tibial tendon insufficiency, diabetic neuropathy, and cerebral palsy. Charnley introduced compression external fixation, which increased rate of fusion.[19] The AO interfragmentary compression principles were used to improve rates of osseous union. Contemporary methods of fixation have increased rates of union further.[20-22] More accurate and safe screw placement is possible with modern equipment.[23] Examples of these include modified blade plates, chevron cuts, bone graft "dowels," and hindfoot intramedullary nails.[21,24,25] Arthroscopically assisted tibiotalar fusion may reduce morbidity further, especially in high-risk populations.[20,26]

ANATOMY AND BIOMECHANICS

The tibiotalar joint is one of the key joints fused in a pantalar arthrodesis. The tibia flares out distally, changing from tubular cortical bone to the metaphyseal cancellous bone. The articular surface of the distal tibia is concave. The posterior lip of the plafond is the anchor point for the posterior part of the inferior tibiofibular syndesmotic ligaments. This prevents posterior translation of the talus. The medial and lateral malleoli are the coronal plane translation constraints. The medial border of the tibia is subcutaneous along its entire length, which makes soft tissues particularly at risk.[27]

The medial soft tissues of note are the superficial deltoid, which originates at the anterior colliculus and inserts into the talus, calcaneus, and navicular. The deep deltoid is the primary medial stabilizer and attaches to the posterior colliculus, which is an intra-articular ligament. The lateral collateral ligament includes the anterior talofibular, posterior talofibular, and fibulocalcaneal ligaments, and serve a role in preventing anterior translation or varus tilt of the tibiotalar joint. The tibiotalar articular surface angle is 93° (valgus), whereas the empirical ankle axis is 83° (varus). The fit of the talus in the mortise is precise and it is the most congruent weightbearing joint. The mortise width changes less than 2 mm throughout the ankle range of motion. Because the ankle axis is oblique there is obligator internal rotation with plantarflexion and external rotation with dorsiflexion.

The subtalar joint is another key joint fused in a pantalar arthrodesis. Articulation is between talus and calcaneus, which are obliquely oriented to each other. The superior surface of the calcaneus has three articular facets: the large posterior facet, and smaller middle and anterior facets. The facets function as a single articulation with the talus. The middle and anterior facets are contiguous and bear more weight per unit area than the posterior facet. The subtalar joint plays a critical role in accommodation of the foot on uneven ground, through inversion and eversion.

The transverse tarsal joint is also fused in a pantalar arthrodesis. The joint complex is also referred to as the Chopart joint and includes the talonavicular and calcaneocuboid joints. It is responsible for the motion between the hindfoot and the midfoot. Anterior portion of the calcaneus articulates with the cuboid creating a mobile unit. The longitudinal axis of the talus deviates 35° medially from the lateral aspect of the calcaneus such that the talar head lies medial and proximal to the calcaneocuboid joint, and the talar head articulates with the navicular and is connected by the spring ligament. These two articulations also correspond to the two columns of the foot, the stiff medial column, and the mobile lateral column.

Limited hindfoot arthrodesis (two or fewer joints) alters gait less severely than pantalar arthrodesis.[28] In level gait, major contribution to motion in sagittal plane is tibiotalar joint. Fusion at the ankle reduces dorsiflexion by half and plantarflexion by 70% with an overall 10% increase in energy expenditure. Fusion reduces coronal plane motion by 30% when ankle arthrodesis is performed. In comparison, triple arthrodesis results in 12% to 15% decrease in sagittal plane motion, and coronal plane motion decreased by 60% secondary to subtalar portion of arthrodesis. Restricted coronal plane motion is well tolerated in level gait and on flat surfaces.

PREOPERATIVE PLANNING

All patients are evaluated in clinic with documentation of patient history, clinical examination, and radiographic evaluation of the limb. Radiographs of the ankle (anteroposterior, mortise, and lateral) and radiographs of the foot (anteroposterior, internal oblique, external oblique, and lateral) are obtained and evaluated. Computed tomography (CT) of the limb from proximal tibia to foot is obtained for preoperative planning. CT allows for evaluation of bone loss, possible need for staging or additional procedures, and planning of implant placement. Clinical assessment is undertaken in the clinic with a focus on soft tissues, neurologic status, and vascular status. When possible, the contralateral limb is examined to compare the deformed limb with the unaffected side. When significant soft tissue compromise is present, the patient is referred to plastic surgery for consideration of preoperative or concomitant soft tissue management procedure.

OPERATIVE PROCEDURE

Pantalar arthrodesis is a procedure that is accomplished with various fixation strategies, including plate and screw fixation, staples, intramedullary device, and external fixation. Here we highlight the procedural notes for three such strategies. Notably, patient positioning and preparation are similar for all three procedures.

Patient Preparation and Positioning

The patient is positioned supine on a radiolucent operating table. Either a spinal or general anesthesia is used. A sandbag or folded surgical drape is placed under the buttock of the affected limb to internally rotate it and bring the lateral aspect of ankle into view. The limb is prepared and draped free. A tourniquet is applied for use as needed.

Approach and Joint Preparation

An L-shaped skin incision is made using a #15 blade. The incision starts 7 cm proximal and posterior to tip of the lateral malleolus and is curved distally and anteriorly 5 cm beyond tip of malleolus. This minimizes disturbance of inferior ligaments of the talus and preserves its blood supply. Superficial dissection encounters the peroneal tendons, which are released from their sheath and displaced inferiorly. The tendons are divided if necessary to correct deformity. Further dissection encounters the calcaneofibular ligament, which is sharply divided. Next, the lateral malleolus is osteotomized in a step-cut fashion. The foot is supinated to expose tibiotalar joint. A lamina spreader is used to pry open the joint. The cartilage is denuded to bleeding cancellous bone using a combination of curettes, osteotomes, and ronguers. The joint is fenestrated with a 2–0 drill bit. Next the peroneal tendons are displaced superiorly. The subtalar joint is brought into view by distracting talus proximally and supinating the foot. The subtalar joint cartilage is denuded to subchondral bone using curettes, osteotomes, and rongeurs to the point the flexor hallucis longus tendon on medial side is visible. Next, the peroneal tendons are displaced inferiorly, the talonavicular ligaments are divided, and joint space is distracted. The cartilage is denuded and joint fenestrated with a drill. To correct any varus or valgus deformity, remove the subtalar or midtarsal joint bone to obtain plantigrade foot. The calcaneocuboid joint is opened, and cartilage is denuded and fenestrated with a drill. At this point, all four joint surfaces are prepared for fusion. If neutral dorsiflexion is not achieved by the previously mentioned procedures, a Hoke Achilles tenotomy is performed percutaneously using three separate incisions posteriorly using an #11 blade. The foot and ankle should then be positioned, with the ankle in neutral dorsiflexion, slight valgus, and slight external rotation.

Fixation with Intramedullary Device and Independent Screws

A hindfoot nail provides adequate fixation and results in reliable fusion.[29] Start by placing a threaded guidewire up through the heel across the tibiotalar joint, subtalar joint, and into the tibia under fluoroscopic guidance. A started drill bit is used to create a tract for the nail. Ream the tibial canal until there is chatter. Measure the appropriate length of nail required and choose nail diameter 1 mm less than the final reamer size. Wounds are then thoroughly irrigated, and the nail is placed with one distal interlocking bolt placed in the dynamization hole. Next, the calcaneal interlocking bolt is placed. Then compress using the screwdriver, and final position of the nail and compression of prepared joints is confirmed under fluoroscopy. Then place the remaining calcaneal and subtalar joint interlocking bolts. Morselized bone graft obtained from debridement is used as an augment for the talonavicular joint. This joint is internally fixed next using two 3.5 fully threaded screws placed across the joint, one medial and one dorsal. Alternatively, the talonavicular joint is internally fixed with a single large frag cannulated screw or a staple.

The fibula is repaired by debriding the soft tissues from the talar tibial side and then burred off the fibular side, with the fibula positioned into its fibular groove and two 4.5 screws holding it in place.

Fixation with Independent Cannulated Screws

A series of 5.0 to 8.0 partially threaded screws are used to stabilize the hindfoot and ankle after joint preparation as previously mentioned.[30] A single cannulated screw from the heel across the subtalar joint stabilizes the subtalar joint. Two additional screws are placed anteromedial into the lateral talar shoulder and posterolateral in the interval between the fibula and Achilles tendon from the tibia into the talar neck.

A supplementary screw across the subtalar and tibiotalar joint is an option. The transverse tarsal joint is positioned in neutral pronation-supination and plantigrade and held in position with Kirschner wires. Talonavicular joint is fixed with one or two 5.0 cannulated screws placed retrograde from the navicular to the talus. The calcaneocuboid joint is fixed with cannulated screw or staple.

External Fixation with Ilizarov Apparatus

The Ilizarov apparatus is a strategy typically reserved for revision surgery in the setting of nonunion.[31,32] If a hindfoot nail is present, the interlocking bolts and nail are removed using prior incisions. Independent cancellous screws can also be removed using small percutaneous incisions. Fluoroscopy is used to make skin markings at the level of nonunion. A longitudinal lateral incision is made midline to the fibula and the fibula is exposed. An acetabular reamer is used to ream the fibula, lateral wall of the talus, and lateral tibial cortex. Next a small osteotomy is used to create a flat surface along the lateral aspect of the fibula. Autograft from the fibular reaming is saved. The fibula is resected or maintained by preserving its posterior soft tissue attachments. Alternatively, a midline incision is used. The articular surfaces are prepared as discussed previously. The position of the prepared joints is temporarily fixed using 2.5 mm Kirschner wires. Ilizarov composite fixator is applied using a two-fold full ring construct. Alternatively, a single full ring and a 5/8 ring is used to prevent soft tissue impingement. Olive wires pins are then placed in the calcaneus. Pin placement in the talus and calcaneus is restricted to the safe zone, being mindful of the neurovascular bundles to be avoided. Avoid transfixation of the distal fibula. Three Kirschner wires are used to fix the distal ring level, which should be placed into the calcaneus. The wires are tensioned to the ring construct to 90 Nm. If the proximal ring is used, it is fixed with two wires into the distal tibia as previously mentioned.

RECOVERY AND REHABILITATION

Patients treated with internal fixation are admitted postoperatively for pain control and intravenous antibiotic prophylaxis. The patient is evaluated in the clinic 10 to 14 days postoperatively for splint removal, wound evaluation, and removal of sutures. Patients remain nonweightbearing for 10 to 12 weeks, mobilizing with a walker or crutches. All patients progress to partial weightbearing starting at 10 to 12 weeks and to full weightbearing on a progressive weightbearing protocol (increasing 25% weightbearing weekly until at full weightbearing). Evaluation in clinic with radiographs is at the 6-week and 12-week postoperative visit. Patients typically transition to athletic shoes starting 12 weeks postoperatively. For patients treated with external fixation, patients are nonweightbearing for 6 to 12 weeks. If the patient was placed in an external fixator, pin care instructions are discussed with the patient preoperatively. Removal of the external fixator occurs at 12 weeks postoperatively.

MANAGEMENT
Immediate Postoperative Management of Pantalar Arthrodesis

Factors affecting longer hospital stay include requiring postoperative admission to an extended care facility, Medicare or Medicaid insurance, treatment with external fixation, diabetic neuropathy, and presence of infection.[33] Multimodal analgesia protocols have been shown to be superior to a traditional opioid-reliant protocol. In a study of 220 patients, those who received a multimodal pain protocol (compromised of opioids, celecoxib, pregabalin, acetaminophen, and prednisone) had shorter hospital stays.[34]

Managing Nonunion with Vascularized Fibular Grafts

Achieving pantalar arthrodesis union in patients with large bone defects is challenging because of the limited amount of surrounding soft tissues. Vascularized fibular grafts are one option in patients with nonunion, large bony defects, or sequelae of infection treated with antibiotic-impregnated cement spacers. One strategy is to use vascularized fibular grafts as a biologic augment. Yajima and colleagues[35] report a case series of seven patients using compression arthrodesis with vascularized fibula grafts resulted in radiographic union in 6 months for six of seven patients. Patients resumed walking without braces in 6 to 20 months. Haddock and colleagues[36] report a retrospective review of vascular bone grafts used in a wide array of foot and ankle reconstruction found all 12 patients achieved union and return to ambulation with full weightbearing.

Managing Nonunion with the Ilizarov Apparatus

Ilizarov fixation is another modality that is used to address failed arthrodesis in the hindfoot. In a case series, 21 patients treated with Ilizarov for nonunion after primary arthrodesis were treated in an Ilizarov apparatus. All patients had a successful union.[31]

OUTCOMES

The outcomes following pantalar arthrodesis have been assessed in several small series. In a study from 2000, of 14 patients undergoing salvage treatment with pantalar arthrodesis, 10 achieved union. Eleven patients had a primary diagnosis of rheumatoid arthritis. Fixation strategy ranged from screws (seven) to external fixator with staples (five), to blade plate (one).[37] In a study comparing pantalar fusion or tibiotalocalcaneal fusion to below knee amputation, there was no statistically significant difference in functional outcomes, satisfactions, or rates of complications.[38]

Outcomes in the posttraumatic and Charcot joints have also been studied. In a study of 12 patients with hindfoot posttraumatic arthritis and eight patients with Charcot arthropathy (type II or IIIA), patients were treated with pantalar arthrodesis. All patients achieved union in a mean of 44 weeks with full weightbearing in 25 weeks. Ten (50%) patients experienced complications, of which four required an additional surgery. No patient received an amputation.[39]

Outcomes in patients with rheumatoid arthritis were reported in a small series from 2011. Involvement of the hindfoot in rheumatoid arthritis ranges from 46% to 90%. A case series of 17 patients with inflammatory pantalar arthritis treated with pantalar arthrodesis resulted in significant improvements in pain scores, functional outcome scores (Short Form-12), and overall high level of patient satisfaction.[40]

Patients with paralytic foot deformities also have overall satisfactory outcomes following treatment with pantalar arthrodesis. Pantalar arthrodesis is considered a final salvage option for patients with paralytic foot deformities. Twenty-four patients underwent one-stage arthrodesis for sequelae of poliomyelitis. Eleven of 24 patients experienced complications including wound healing issues (nine) and infections (two). Overall patients had satisfactory outcomes with good Short Form-36 scores.[29]

The most common complication following primary ankle arthrodesis is ankle nonunion, with a rate as high as 30%. Rates of other complications following pantalar arthrodesis including malunion, infection, osteoarthritis of adjacent joints, neurovascular injury, and wound-healing problems are as high as 60%.[41] A single case report of occlusion of the posterior tibial artery after pantalar arthrodesis was reported in 2007. The authors attributed the arterial occlusion to stretching and impingement of the posterior tibial artery over the posterior talar process. The authors were able to diagnose the occlusion using intraoperative Doppler ultrasound.[42]

CASE STUDIES
Case #1

A 67-year-old man was first evaluated in our clinic for bilateral clubfoot deformity status postcircumferential releases in the 1950s. He had a normal childhood and participated in sports activities and did well until age 50, when he underwent an uninstrumented ankle fusion for right ankle arthritis. He returned to walking and skiing after the surgery. A few years before our clinic evaluation, he began to have anterolateral ankle pain managed nonoperatively. The pain since has advanced and prevents him from standing, walking, and participating in desired activities. His past medical history includes myocardial infarct status post stent placement at age 50 and history of hepatitis C treated with medication therapy.

On examination he was found to have wasting of the gastric-soleus complex, varus hindfoot alignment, and tenderness to palpation about the sinus tarsi and lateral ankle. He had no ankle range of motion and minimal subtalar joint range of motion. The midfoot was found to be stiff including the first, fourth, and fifth rays. He had normal sensation, motor function, and vasculature of the foot.

Radiographs demonstrated equinus positioning of the ankle, tibiotalar joint arthrodesis, significant arthrosis of the hindfoot and talonavicular joint, and mild midfoot arthritis. He had a decreased kite talocalcaneal angle consistent with varus alignment. CT imaging revealed only partial union of the ankle fusion. He was counseled regarding the nature of the condition and the patient elected to proceed with pantalar fusion (**Figs. 1** and **2**).

Arthrodesis of the subtalar and tibiotalar joints was conducted using the Wright Medical (Memphis, TN) VALOR nail. Arthrodesis of the lateral aspect of the calcaneocuboid joint used the claw plate. Arthrodesis of the talonavicular joint was completed using two 5.0 cannulated screws. In addition, 15 mL of cancellous bone allograft was used (**Fig. 3**).

The patient was admitted to the hospital for intravenous antibiotics and pain control postoperatively. He was initially placed in a splint and transitioned to a CAM boot at 2 weeks postoperatively. He maintained nonweightbearing status for 3 months, at which time he began a protocol of progressive weightbearing. At 3 months postoperatively, he was evaluated with radiographs demonstrating consolidation of the sites of arthrodesis with intact implants.

Case #2

A 67-year-old man with a history of bilateral total ankle arthroplasties was evaluated in our clinic. He had a revision left total ankle arthroplasty in 2014 with conversion to an

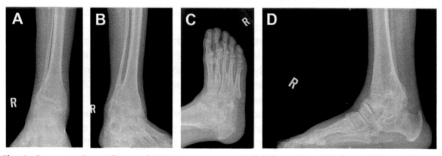

Fig. 1. Preoperative radiographs anteroposterior (AP) (*A*), mortise (*B*), foot oblique (*C*), and lateral (*D*) demonstrating deformity.

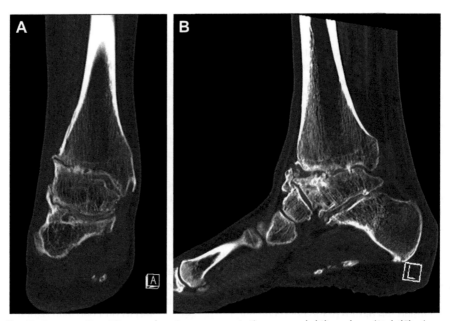

Fig. 2. Preoperative CT scan showing representative coronal (*A*) and sagittal (*B*) views demonstrating extent of joint destruction.

INBONE II prosthesis (Wright Medical). He noted he began having intermittent swelling and activity-related pain in the left ankle while he was rehabilitating from a right total knee arthroplasty. The pain advanced to the point of interfering with daily activities and diminishing his quality of life. Of note, he had a past medical history including Crohn disease and obesity with a body mass index of 32 and a past surgical history, which includes right total hip arthroplasty, right total knee arthroplasty, and left total shoulder arthroplasty in addition to bilateral total ankle arthroplasties.

On examination he was found to have a plantigrade foot with moderate swelling about the ankle and multiple well-healed incisions. He was globally tender to palpation about the ankle. His ankle range of motion was painful from neutral dorsiflexion and 20° of plantarflexion.

Radiographs demonstrated left ankle interval subsidence of the talar component with heterotopic ossification about the medial, posterior, and anterior ankle. In addition, the tibial component appeared in stable position without osteolysis (**Fig. 4**).

The patient was initially treated nonoperatively with IDEO brace. Surgical management was discussed including fusion and below knee amputation. The patient elected to proceed with a pantalar arthrodesis.

He underwent removal of ankle arthroplasty implant and arthrodesis of subtalar and tibiotalar joint with Wright Medical VALOR nail. Arthrodesis of the talonavicular joint was accomplished with a DePuy Synthes (Raynham, MA) BME compression staple and 3.5-mm cortical screw. In addition, femoral head allograft and 25 mL of DePuy Synthes Invivogen biologics was used (**Fig. 5**).

The patient was admitted to the hospital postoperatively for intravenous antibiotics and pain control. He maintained nonweightbearing status for a total of 3 months. He was started on a standard progressive weightbearing program at that time. At his last follow-up, he was found to be free of complications, progression of arthrodesis consolidation on radiographs, and pain well controlled.

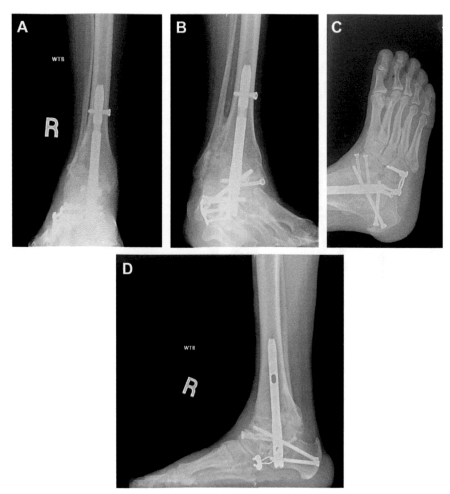

Fig. 3. Postoperative radiographs (12 weeks) AP (*A*), mortise (*B*), foot oblique (*C*), and lateral (*D*) demonstrating pantalar arthrodesis fixation.

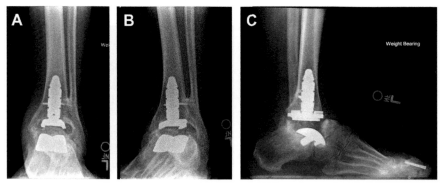

Fig. 4. Preoperative radiographs AP (*A*), mortise (*B*), and lateral (*C*) demonstrating failure of talar implant.

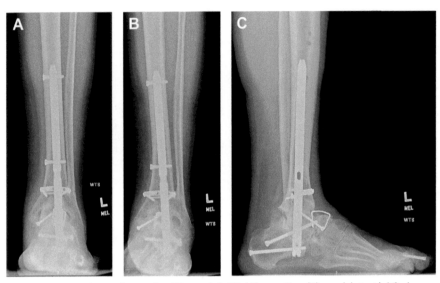

Fig. 5. Postoperative radiographs (12 weeks) AP (*A*), mortise (*B*), and lateral (*C*) demonstrating arthrodesis pantalar fixation.

Case #3

A 67-year-old man had left Charcot ankle and foot secondary to poorly controlled type 2 diabetes mellitus with varus ankle deformity with chronic peroneal tendon rupture. He developed atraumatic chronic skin breakdown over the fibula with subsequent infection. Osteomyelitis was subsequently treated with standard long-term intravenous antibiotics. He underwent multiple rounds of intravenous antibiotics for recurrent infection with methicillin-susceptible *Staphylococcus aureus*, including hyperbaric chamber treatments of the chronic ulcerations. The patient had undergone treatment for more than 1 year before presentation in our clinic. The patient has a past surgical history that includes a left calcaneal osteotomy to correct congenital varus deformity (**Fig. 6**).

The patient was treated with a two-stage procedure. The first procedure involved partial excision of the infected bone of fibula and medial release with posterior tibial tendon lengthening. He then underwent pantalar arthrodesis of the subtalar and tibio-talar joints with the Wright Medical VALOR nail. Arthrodesis of the calcaneocuboid

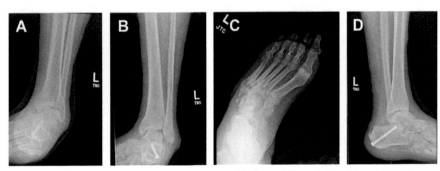

Fig. 6. Preoperative radiographs AP (*A*), mortise (*B*), foot oblique (*C*), and lateral (*D*) demonstrating deformity present.

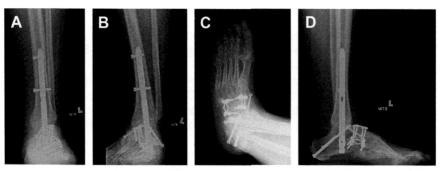

Fig. 7. Postoperative radiographs (12 weeks) AP (*A*), mortise (*B*), foot oblique (*C*), and lateral (*D*) demonstrating pantalar arthrodesis fixation.

joint was achieved with the Wright medical claw plates. In addition, 3 mL of cancellous bone allograft was used as an augment (**Fig. 7**).

Postoperatively he remained nonweightbearing for a total of 3 months. He was transitioned from a cast to a CAM boot at 6 weeks postoperatively. He began a protocol of progressive weightbearing at 3 months postoperatively. At his final clinic follow-up at 21 months, he had no complications, reported no pain, and was ambulatory with a rocker-bottom shoe. He continued work as a physical therapist and was overall satisfied with his postoperative course.

SUMMARY

A triple arthrodesis is comprised of subtalar, talonavicular, and calcaneocuboid joints arthrodesis. The goal of the procedure is to obtain a correction of deformity and achieve a plantigrade, functional, painless, stable, weightbearing foot that can be used to ambulate. There are several approaches and fixation strategies that result in successful clinical union and should be chosen to match the clinical situation. Modern techniques result in high rates of union and pain relief.

CLINICS CARE POINTS

- Pantalar arthrodesis is a surgical option to provide a stable base for weightbearing in patients with severe deformity and arthritis of the ankle, subtalar, and Chopart joints.
- During initial clinical assessment of the patient's soft tissues, if there is significant soft tissue compromise, we recommend referral to plastic surgery for evaluation of preoperative or concomitant soft tissue management.
- When using independent cannulated screws for fixation, we recommend partially threaded screws 5.0 mm to 8.0 mm. It is important to position the transverse tarsal joint in neutral pronation-supination and plantigrade. Use Kirschner wires to hold its position provisionally before fixation with screws.
- Although modern techniques offer high rates of success for pantalar arthrodesis, it is important to counsel patients that the goal of surgery is limited to achieving a painless, plantigrade, and stable foot.

DISCLOSURE

S. Chawla has nothing to disclose.

REFERENCES

1. Stone MA, Flato RR, Pannell W, et al. Operatively treated talus fractures: complications and survivorship in a large patient sample. J Foot Ankle Surg 2018;57(4): 737–41.
2. LaClair SM. Reconstruction of the varus ankle from soft-tissue procedures with osteotomy through arthrodesis. Foot Ankle Clin 2007;12(1):153–76, x.
3. Ellington JK, Myerson MS. Surgical correction of the ball and socket ankle joint in the adult associated with a talonavicular tarsal coalition. Foot Ankle Int 2013; 34(10):1381–8.
4. Dhillon MS, Agashe V, Patil SD. Role of surgery in management of osteo-articular tuberculosis of the foot and ankle. Open Orthop J 2017;11:633–50.
5. Hoke M. An operation for stabilizing paralytic feet. JBJS 1921;3(10):494–507.
6. Hunt JC, Brooks AL. Subtalar extra-articular arthrodesis for correction of paralytic valgus deformity of the foot: evaluation of forty-four procedures with particular reference to associated tendon transference. JBJS 1965;47(7):1310–4.
7. Lambrinudi C. New operation on drop-foot. Br J Surg 1927;15(58):193–200.
8. Lance EM, Paval A, Fries I, et al. Arthrodesis of the ankle joint: a follow-up study. Clin Orthopaedics Relat Research® 1979;(142):146–58.
9. Whitman R. The operative treatment of paralytic talipes of the calcaneus type. 1. Am J Med Sci (1827-1924) 1901;122(6):593.
10. Ansart MB. Pan-arthrodesis for paralytic flail foot. J Bone Joint Surg Br 1951; 33(4):503–7.
11. Campbell W. Bone-block operation for drop-foot; analysis of end results. JBJS 1930;12(2):317–24.
12. Cook AG, Stern WG, Ryerson EW. Report of the commission appointed by the American Orthopedic Association for the study of stabilizing operations on the foot. JBJS 1923;5(1):135–40.
13. Marek FM, Schein AJ. Aseptic necrosis of the astragalus following arthrodesing procedures of the tarsus. JBJS 1945;27(4):587–94.
14. Pyevich MT, Saltzman CL, Callaghan JJ, et al. Total ankle arthroplasty: a unique design. Two to twelve-year follow-up. JBJS 1998;80(10):1410–20.
15. Wetmore RS, Drennan J. Long-term results of triple arthrodesis in Charcot-Marie-Tooth disease. J Bone Joint Surg Am 1989;71(3):417–22.
16. Jones R. An operation for paralytic calcaneo-cavus. JBJS 1908;2(4):371–6.
17. RYERSON EW. Arthrodesing operations on the feet. JBJS 1923;5(3):453–71.
18. Staples OS. Posterior arthrodesis of the ankle and subtalar joints. JBJS 1956; 38(1):50–83.
19. Pfahler M, Krödel A, Tritschler A, et al. Role of internal and external fixation in ankle fusion. Arch Orthop Trauma Surg 1996;115(3–4):146–8.
20. O'Brien TS, Hart TS, Shereff MJ, et al. Open versus arthroscopic ankle arthrodesis: a comparative study. Foot Ankle Int 1999;20(6):368–74.
21. Quill G. Tibiotalocalcaneal and pantalar arthrodesis. Foot Ankle Clin 1996;1(1): 199–210.
22. Sowa DT, Krackow KA. Ankle fusion: a new technique of internal fixation using a compression blade plate. Foot & ankle 1989;9(5):232–40.
23. Gable SJ, Bohay DR, Manoli A. Aiming guide for accurate placement of subtalar joint screws. Foot Ankle Int 1995;16(4):238–9.
24. Kelikian AS. Operative treatment of the foot and ankle. New York, NY: McGraw-Hill Professional Publishing; 1999.

25. Kile TA, Donnelly RE, Gehrke JC, et al. Tibiotalocalcaneal arthrodesis with an intramedullary device. Foot Ankle Int 1994;15(12):669–73.
26. Turan I, Wredmark T, Felländer-Tsai L. Arthroscopic ankle arthrodesis in rheumatoid arthritis. Clin Orthop Relat Res 1995;320:110–4.
27. Browner BD, Jupiter J, Krettek C, et al. Skeletal trauma e-book. Philadelphia, PA: Elsevier Health Sciences; 2014.
28. Faillace JJ, Leopold SS, Brage ME. Extended hindfoot fusions and pantalar fusions. History, biomechanics, and clinical results. Foot Ankle Clin 2000;5(4): 777–98.
29. Provelengios S, Papavasiliou KA, Kyrkos MJ, et al. The role of pantalar arthrodesis in the treatment of paralytic foot deformities. Surgical technique. J Bone Joint Surg Am 2010;92(Suppl 1 Pt 1):44–54.
30. Cooper PS. Pantalar Arthrodesis Tech Orthopaedics 2000;15(3):252–8.
31. Khodadadyan-Klostermann C, Raschke M, Mittlmeier T, et al. Ankle and pan-talar arthrodesis with Ilizarov composite hybrid fixation: operative technique and review of 21 cases. Foot Ankle Surg 2001;7(3):149–56.
32. Paley D, Lamm BM, Katsenis D, et al. Treatment of malunion and nonunion at the site of an ankle fusion with the Ilizarov apparatus. Surgical technique. J Bone Joint Surg Am 2006;88(Suppl 1 Pt 1):119–34.
33. Deister J, Cothern BG, Williams C, et al. Factors predicting length of hospital stay and extended care facility admission after hindfoot arthrodesis procedures. J Foot Ankle Surg 2017;56(4):805–12.
34. Michelson JD, Addante RA, Charlson MD. Multimodal analgesia therapy reduces length of hospitalization in patients undergoing fusions of the ankle and hindfoot. Foot Ankle Int 2013;34(11):1526–34.
35. Yajima H, Kobata Y, Tomita Y, et al. Ankle and pantalar arthrodeses using vascularized fibular grafts. Foot Ankle Int 2004;25(1):3–7.
36. Haddock NT, Wapner K, Levin LS. Vascular bone transfer options in the foot and ankle: a retrospective review and update on strategies. Plast Reconstr Surg 2013; 132(3):685–93.
37. Acosta R, Ushiba J, Cracchiolo A 3rd. The results of a primary and staged pantalar arthrodesis and tibiotalocalcaneal arthrodesis in adult patients. Foot Ankle Int 2000;21(3):182–94.
38. Oswal C, Patel S, Malhotra K, et al. Limb salvage versus below knee amputation for severe adult lower limb deformity: a retrospective, comparative series. Foot Ankle Surg 2021. https://doi.org/10.1016/j.fas.2021.07.001.
39. Herscovici D, Sammarco GJ, Sammarco VJ, et al. Pantalar arthrodesis for posttraumatic arthritis and diabetic neuroarthropathy of the ankle and hindfoot. Foot Ankle Int 2011;32(6):581–8.
40. McKinley JC, Shortt N, Arthur C, et al. Outcomes following pantalar arthrodesis in rheumatoid arthritis. Foot Ankle Int 2011;32(7):681–5.
41. Frey C, Halikus NM, Vu-Rose T, et al. A review of ankle arthrodesis: predisposing factors to nonunion. Foot Ankle Int 1994;15(11):581–4.
42. Tauladan J, Koedam NA, Rijcken THP, et al. Occlusion of the posterior tibial artery after pantalar arthrodesis: a case report. Acta Orthopaedica 2007;78(3):442–3.

UNITED STATES POSTAL SERVICE®
Statement of Ownership, Management, and Circulation (All Periodicals Publications Except Requester Publications)

1. Publication Title	2. Publication Number	3. Filing Date
FOOT AND ANKLE CLINICS OF NORTH AMERICA	016 – 368	9/18/2022

4. Issue Frequency	5. Number of Issues Published Annually	6. Annual Subscription Price
MAR, JUN, SEP, DEC	4	$351.00

7. Complete Mailing Address of Known Office of Publication (Not printer) (Street, city, county, state, and ZIP+4®)

ELSEVIER INC.
230 Park Avenue, Suite 800
New York, NY 10169

Contact Person
Malathi Samayan
Telephone (Include area code)
91-44-4299-4507

8. Complete Mailing Address of Headquarters or General Business Office of Publisher (Not printer)

ELSEVIER INC.
230 Park Avenue, Suite 800
New York, NY 10169

9. Full Names and Complete Mailing Addresses of Publisher, Editor, and Managing Editor (Do not leave blank)

Publisher (Name and complete mailing address)

DOLORES MELONI, ELSEVIER INC.
1600 JOHN F KENNEDY BLVD. SUITE 1800
PHILADELPHIA, PA 19103-2899

Editor (Name and complete mailing address)

Megan Ashdown, ELSEVIER INC.
1600 JOHN F KENNEDY BLVD. SUITE 1800
PHILADELPHIA, PA 19103-2899

Managing Editor (Name and complete mailing address)

PATRICK MANLEY, ELSEVIER INC.
1600 JOHN F KENNEDY BLVD. SUITE 1800
PHILADELPHIA, PA 19103-2899

10. Owner (Do not leave blank. If the publication is owned by a corporation, give the name and address of the corporation immediately followed by the names and addresses of all stockholders owning or holding 1 percent or more of the total amount of stock. If not owned by a corporation, give the names and addresses of the individual owners. If owned by a partnership or other unincorporated firm, give its name and address as well as those of each individual owner. If the publication is published by a nonprofit organization, give its name and address.)

Full Name	Complete Mailing Address
WHOLLY OWNED SUBSIDIARY OF REED/ELSEVIER, US HOLDINGS	1600 JOHN F KENNEDY BLVD. SUITE 1800 PHILADELPHIA, PA 19103-2899

11. Known Bondholders, Mortgagees, and Other Security Holders Owning or Holding 1 Percent or More of Total Amount of Bonds, Mortgages, or Other Securities. If none, check box ► ☐ None

Full Name	Complete Mailing Address
N/A	

12. Tax Status (For completion by nonprofit organizations authorized to mail at nonprofit rates) (Check one)
The purpose, function, and nonprofit status of this organization and the exempt status for federal income tax purposes:
☒ Has Not Changed During Preceding 12 Months
☐ Has Changed During Preceding 12 Months (Publisher must submit explanation of change with this statement)

PS Form 3526, July 2014 (Page 1 of 4 (see instructions page 4)) PSN: 7530-01-000-9931   PRIVACY NOTICE: See our privacy policy on www.usps.com.

---

13. Publication Title	14. Issue Date for Circulation Data Below
FOOT AND ANKLE CLINICS OF NORTH AMERICA	JUNE 2022

15. Extent and Nature of Circulation			Average No. Copies Each Issue During Preceding 12 Months	No. Copies of Single Issue Published Nearest to Filing Date
a. Total Number of Copies (Net press run)			266	232
b. Paid Circulation (By Mail and Outside the Mail)	(1)	Mailed Outside-County Paid Subscriptions Stated on PS Form 3541 (Include paid distribution above nominal rate, advertiser's proof copies, and exchange copies)	160	150
	(2)	Mailed In-County Paid Subscriptions Stated on PS Form 3541 (Include paid distribution above nominal rate, advertiser's proof copies, and exchange copies)	0	0
	(3)	Paid Distribution Outside the Mails Including Sales Through Dealers and Carriers, Street Vendors, Counter Sales, and Other Paid Distribution Outside USPS®	78	65
	(4)	Paid Distribution by Other Classes of Mail Through the USPS (e.g., First-Class Mail®)	0	0
c. Total Paid Distribution (Sum of 15b (1), (2), (3), and (4))		►	238	215
d. Free or Nominal Rate Distribution (By Mail and Outside the Mail)	(1)	Free or Nominal Rate Outside-County Copies included on PS Form 3541	13	3
	(2)	Free or Nominal Rate In-County Copies Included on PS Form 3541	0	0
	(3)	Free or Nominal Rate Copies Mailed at Other Classes Through the USPS (e.g., First-Class Mail)	0	0
	(4)	Free or Nominal Rate Distribution Outside the Mail (Carriers or other means)	0	0
e. Total Free or Nominal Rate Distribution (Sum of 15d (1), (2), (3) and (4))		►	13	3
f. Total Distribution (Sum of 15c and 15e)		►	251	218
g. Copies not Distributed (See instructions to Publishers #4 (page #3))		►	15	14
h. Total (Sum of 15f and g)		►	266	232
i. Percent Paid (15c divided by 15f times 100)		►	94.82%	98.62%

* If you are claiming electronic copies, go to line 16 on page 3. If you are not claiming electronic copies, skip to line 17 on page 3.

16. Electronic Copy Circulation	Average No. Copies Each Issue During Preceding 12 Months	No. Copies of Single Issue Published Nearest to Filing Date
a. Paid Electronic Copies ►		
b. Total Paid Print Copies (Line 15c) + Paid Electronic Copies (Line 16a) ►		
c. Total Print Distribution (Line 15f) + Paid Electronic Copies (Line 16a) ►		
d. Percent Paid (Both Print & Electronic Copies) (16b divided by 16c × 100) ►		

☒ I certify that 50% of all my distributed copies (electronic and print) are paid above a nominal price.

17. Publication of Statement of Ownership
☒ If the publication is a general publication, publication of this statement is required. Will be printed ☐ Publication not required.
in the DECEMBER 2022 issue of this publication.

18. Signature and Title of Editor, Publisher, Business Manager, or Owner

Malathi Samayan - Distribution Controller

Malathi Samayan   Date 9/18/2022

I certify that all information furnished on this form is true and complete. I understand that anyone who furnishes false or misleading information on this form or who omits material or information requested on the form may be subject to criminal sanctions (including fines and imprisonment) and/or civil sanctions (including civil penalties).

PS Form 3526, July 2014 (Page 3 of 4)   PRIVACY NOTICE: See our privacy policy on www.usps.com.

Moving?

Make sure your subscription moves with you!

To notify us of your new address, find your **Clinics Account Number** (located on your mailing label above your name), and contact customer service at:

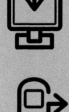

Email: journalscustomerservice-usa@elsevier.com

800-654-2452 (subscribers in the U.S. & Canada)
314-447-8871 (subscribers outside of the U.S. & Canada)

Fax number: 314-447-8029

Elsevier Health Sciences Division
Subscription Customer Service
3251 Riverport Lane
Maryland Heights, MO 63043

*To ensure uninterrupted delivery of your subscription, please notify us at least 4 weeks in advance of move.

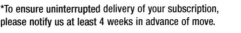

9780323849463